Injectable
Contraceptives

Injectable Contraceptives

Their role in family planning care

WORLD HEALTH ORGANIZATION
GENEVA
1990

WHO Library Cataloguing in Publication Data

Injectable contraceptives : their role in family planning care.

1. Contraceptive agents, Female   2. Delayed-action preparations
3. Family planning   4. Program evaluation

ISBN 92 4 154402 3   (NLM Classification: QV 177)

© World Health Organization 1990

TYPESET IN INDIA
PRINTED IN ENGLAND
87/7490—Macmillan/Clays/GCW—8000

Contents

Preface

The growing interest in and demand for injectable contraceptives in many parts of the world led to the publication by WHO in 1982 of *Injectable hormonal contraceptives: technical and safety aspects* (WHO Offset Publication No. 65). The developments in the field and the experience gained in the management of family planning programmes, and in particular in the use of injectable contraceptives since that date, have made it necessary to produce the present revised and updated version of that publication. This is all the more important since, as an effective family planning method, injectable contraceptives can make an important contribution to the protection of the health of mother and child. They are compatible with the primary health care strategy, so that both the accessibility and awareness of birth spacing can be increased, since a larger number of people can be reached than would ordinarily be possible through the formal health care system.

The primary purpose of these guidelines is to assist those responsible for the development and management of family planning and health programmes in introducing or increasing the availability of injectable contraceptives. They are designed to serve the needs of various categories of health personnel, including programme managers, administrators and service providers. Essential technical information about injectables, their effects and related medical issues is included, so as to ensure that such personnel have the necessary understanding of this method of contraception. The guidelines also contain information of practical value to those initiating programmes. Thus, chapters on organizing, managing and evaluating a programme are included, together with an annex containing a model patient record form that can be adapted for use in particular settings.

The important contributions of Dr Viopapa Annandale, United Kingdom, Dr B. Affandi, Indonesia, Dr I. S. Fraser, Australia, Ms J. Hutchings, PATH, USA, Dr P. Senanayake, IPPF, United Kingdom, as well as of the members of the Task Force on Long-Acting Systemic Agents for Fertility Regulation of the Special Programme of Research, Development and Research Training in Human Reproduction, and of the many reviewers who have given unselfishly of their time in the preparation of this text, are gratefully acknowledged.

WHO is most grateful to the United Nations Population Fund (UNFPA) for its financial contribution towards the preparation and publication of this document.

Comments and queries on this publication should be addressed to: Maternal and Child Health, World Health Organization, 1211 Geneva 27, Switzerland.

1. Background information and programme considerations

Development of injectable contraceptives

Shortly after oral hormonal contraceptives were introduced, it was discovered that the availability of these hormones in the body could be prolonged by adding on an additional chemical group to form an ester. When injected intramuscularly, these compounds are slowly released into the circulation, and thereby provide long-lasting hormonal activity.

Between 1953 and 1957, a considerable number of esters of different estrogens and progestogens were synthesized. Some of these could be formulated only as oily solutions, whereas others could be made up as microcrystalline suspensions. The two that have come to be the most widely used as injectable contraceptives are depot-medroxyprogesterone acetate (DMPA) (a microcrystalline suspension) and norethisterone enantate (NET-EN) (an oily solution).

DMPA was first used in humans in 1960 for the prevention of premature labour and for the treatment of threatened abortion, endometriosis and endometrial carcinoma. It was then sometimes given in doses as high as 1–4 g per injection. It was soon recognized that many women who were treated during pregnancy remained infertile for many months afterwards. This led to the recognition of DMPA's contraceptive properties and proper clinical contraceptive trials were started in 1963. Three separate and independent reports appeared in 1966 indicating a very high effectiveness in preventing pregnancy,

1

since when it has become popular as a contraceptive and is now marketed in over 80 countries and territories.

NET-EN has been used as a contraceptive since 1966, although less extensively than DMPA. It has the disadvantages that more frequent injections are required (2-monthly as compared with 3-monthly) and that pregnancy rates are slightly higher. The discontinuation rates due to irregular bleeding are the same for both DMPA and NET-EN, but fewer women discontinue because of amenorrhoea when using NET-EN. It is now marketed in over 30 countries and territories.

It is estimated that more than 30 million women world-wide have used injectable contraceptives and, of these, over 6 million are using them at present. A list of the countries and territories in which DMPA and NET-EN are registered for use as contraceptives is given in Annex 1.

Formulation and mode of action

Injectable hormonal contraceptives, when properly used, are among the most effective methods of contraception available today, and should therefore be considered for inclusion among the family planning methods available at any clinic or other health facility offering an integrated family planning service.

NET-EN is prepared in an oily solution and, after injection, is hydrolysed to the biologically active steroid norethisterone (NET). In contrast, DMPA is formulated as a microcrystalline suspension of known particle size and the medroxyprogesterone acetate released into the circulation is itself biologically active. NET-EN disappears more rapidly from the circulation than DMPA and it is for this reason that it has to be given at shorter intervals.

In preventing pregnancy, both DMPA and NET-EN act essentially by:

—inhibiting ovulation;

—increasing the viscosity of the cervical secretions, thus forming a barrier to spermatozoa (and to many bacteria);

2

—changing the rate of ovum transport through the fallopian tubes;

—making the endometrium less suitable for implantation.

Role of injectable contraceptives in family planning programmes

The results of various studies, including the World Fertility Survey of 1980, indicate that about half of all married women in the world currently do not want any more children but that only a relatively small proportion use any form of contraception, whether modern or traditional. The need, especially for women in the developing countries, for an effective, safe, and reversible method of contraception that does not interfere with lactation, can be administered by non-physicians in remote areas, is totally independent of coitus and does not require specialized facilities or supplies can therefore hardly be overemphasized. However, every approach to fertility control has its advantages and disadvantages. None is suitable for everyone at every time. None is acceptable in every culture. Each of the currently available modern methods of contraception, including oral contraceptives and intrauterine devices (IUDs), has gained acceptance by some couples at certain stages of their reproductive life. For this reason, family planning programmes typically offer a wide range of methods to potential clients. In addition, experience suggests that a wide choice of contraceptive methods encourages acceptance and continued use, while each additional method contributes independently to the overall prevalence of contraceptive use.

Of the various methods of contraception, injectable contraceptives are particularly useful for couples who have completed their families but are not ready to accept sterilization. They are also useful as a method of spacing for couples planning a birth interval of more than 2 years, since fertility return may be delayed by an average of 6 months when the method is discontinued.

Injectables are also particularly suitable for temporary use by women who require maximum protection following immunization against rubella, for partners of men

3

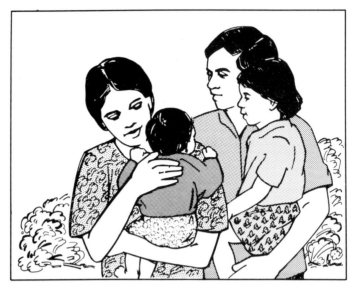

Fig. 1. Injectable contraceptives are suitable for use by couples who do not want any more children, and by those who wish to delay the next pregnancy.

undergoing vasectomy, and for postpartum women awaiting sterilization.

However, the use of long-acting (i.e., effective for two or three months) injectable steroids is associated with menstrual disturbances and a slower return to fertility as compared with IUDs and oral contraceptives. It is also relatively labour-intensive in the sense that health personnel have to provide repeat injections at 2- or 3-monthly intervals, as well as counselling for menstrual disturbances and other minor side-effects. Programme administrators must therefore weigh these disadvantages of injectables against the fact that they provide a long-acting, reversible method of contraception that is totally independent of coital activity, does not require specialized facilities or supplies and can be administered by a non-physician.

Controversy associated with injectable contraceptives

The controversy associated with long-acting hormonal contraceptives has centred around DMPA and the

4

application to market it as a contraceptive in the USA. A major aspect of this controversy has been the interpretation of data from animal toxicology studies, particularly those relating to possible carcinogenic effects. Because of this, numerous reviews have been undertaken by both national and international bodies, the most important of which are summarized below.

In 1978, the Toxicology Review Panel of the WHO Special Programme of Research, Development and Research Training in Human Reproduction, together with other scientists and representatives of six national drug regulatory agencies, reviewed the results of animal and human experiments with DMPA and NET-EN, and concluded that, for DMPA: "The available evidence does not indicate a risk of adverse effects associated with Depo-Provera [DMPA] which would preclude the use of this drug as a contraceptive . . . There is a need to monitor the safety of Depo-Provera on an ongoing basis, and the Special Programme will continue to place high priority on such research."

For NET-EN, the Panel recommended that: "in the light of the findings in the monkey, beagle and rat . . . the current and planned clinical trials of norethisterone enantate should continue."

DMPA was reviewed by the Food and Drug Administration (FDA) in the USA in 1978, and although approval for use as a contraceptive agent was recommended by the FDA's Obstetrics and Gynecology Advisory Committee (a group of specialists who advise the FDA on technical matters), the FDA did not grant such approval.

The International Medical Advisory Panel of the International Planned Parenthood Federation met in 1980 and endorsed the recommendations of WHO, the Ad Hoc Consultative Panel on DMPA of the Agency for International Development, and the Scientific Advisory Committee of the US Food and Drug Administration, that it "continues to be a responsible act of making DMPA available as a contraceptive."

WHO then convened another meeting of experts in 1981,[a] who concluded that:

---

[a] Facts about injectable contraceptives: Memorandum from a WHO Meeting. *Bulletin of the World Health Organization*, **60**: 199–210 (1982).

Injectable contraceptives—both DMPA and NET-EN—offer several advantages as a method of contraception, and have been shown in a number of clinical trials to be effective in preventing pregnancy and acceptable to many women. Although animal data have raised concern about the safety and long-term side-effects of DMPA and NET-EN, certain animal models and the doses used appear not to be appropriate for studying human effects of these steroids. Extensive clinical and epidemiological studies among women using these drugs have thus far demonstrated no life-threatening side-effects.

The most common side-effect is the disturbance of normal menstrual cycles, which occurs in the majority of women using injectable contraception, and is the primary reason for its discontinuation. Women frequently report irregular bleeding, spotting, and amenorrhoea, but heavy or prolonged bleeding is uncommon.

Studies thus far have not shown any serious short- or long-term effects of DMPA or NET-EN. However, both DMPA and NET-EN have been used for a relatively short time, and the potential long-term effects (over more than 15 years) are not yet known.

With regard to metabolic effects, research should continue on the effects and physiological consequences of long-term use of DMPA and NET-EN on carbohydrate and lipid metabolism. In addition, further research is needed regarding the long-term risk of neoplasia among women using DMPA or NET-EN. Finally, the effects on the later development of infants who are exposed to DMPA or NET-EN *in utero* or through breast milk are not known. Research should continue in these areas.

In summary, DMPA and NET-EN appear to be acceptable methods of fertility regulation. Clinical evidence from more than 15 years of use as contraceptive agents shows no additional, and possibly fewer, adverse effects than are found with other hormonal methods of contraception. The particular advantages of DMPA and NET-EN as highly effective, long-lasting and reversible contraceptives make them important as options for women desiring a method of fertility regulation.

Eventually the FDA constituted a Public Board of Inquiry which, in its report of October 1984, stated that the available information on DMPA "does not provide sufficient basis from which FDA can determine that DMPA is safe for general marketing in the United States".

Subsequently the company withdrew its application for marketing.

The concern over DMPA first arose because of the increased incidence of breast cancer it produced in beagle bitches. Animals treated with doses of DMPA ranging from the human equivalent dose to up to 50 times this dosage for periods of up to 7 years developed a larger number of benign and malignant breast nodules than control animals. Since that time, a large amount of data, from both animals and humans, has been accumulated showing the beagle bitch to be a poor model for predicting the risk of breast cancer in humans. For this reason, the United Kingdom Committee for the Safety of Medicines and other drug regulatory bodies in western European countries no longer require the use of this animal model in the toxicology testing of hormonal contraceptives. Since the application for a licence to market DMPA as a contraceptive in the USA was withdrawn, the FDA has reviewed its requirements for testing of steroid hormones, dropping the need for testing in the monkey, and reducing the period of testing in the beagle from 7 to 3 years.

WHO has published the results from an interim analysis of a 3-country case–control study of DMPA and cancer, which included a total of 427 cases of breast cancer and 5951 controls.[a] The relative risk of breast cancer among women who had used DMPA was 1.0, suggesting that no association exists between DMPA use and breast cancer. However, since few women use DMPA for more than 1 or 2 years, it is difficult to draw any firm conclusions about long-term DMPA use and breast cancer.

Concern also arose from animal toxicology studies when a small number of malignant and premalignant endometrial lesions were observed in rhesus monkeys treated with DMPA and NET-EN. Again, there is evidence that these findings are not predictive of a risk of endometrial cancer in humans and, in fact, there is reason to expect that administration of these progestogens will actually reduce the risk of endometrial cancer in women. The interim results from the WHO study mentioned above showed a relative risk of 0.3 for endometrial cancer which, although

---

[a] Depot-medroxyprogesterone acetate (DMPA) and cancer: Memorandum from a WHO Meeting. *Bulletin of the World Health Organization*, **64**: 375–382 (1986).

not statistically significant, does support the hypothesis that use of DMPA might protect women against this form of cancer.

A few published studies have reported a small increased risk of cervical cancer among women who have used DMPA, especially for long periods of time. However, most of these studies have either not included appropriate control groups or have not taken into account the sexual habits of DMPA users or their partners—an important source of bias in virtually all studies of cervical cancer. The largest and most recent study on this subject is a WHO study, in which an attempt has been made to take sexual practices into account. The most recently published analysis shows an overall relative risk of 1.2,[a] which is not significant, suggesting that there is no overall change in the risk of cervical cancer among DMPA users. Furthermore, the risk did not seem to increase with length of use of DMPA. However, it must again be emphasized that long-term use of DMPA is uncommon and it is thus not possible to state categorically that there is no increased risk with long-term use.

Two other cancers have been studied with respect to DMPA—ovarian cancer and liver cancer—but neither has been found with increased frequency among women who have used it. There are no data from human studies on NET-EN and cancer risk as too short a time has elapsed since the number of users became large enough to allow meaningful studies to be conducted.

Factors affecting availability and acceptance

Many factors affect the availability and acceptance of injectable contraceptives, but the availability will depend largely on the interest and commitment of the health professionals concerned, who in turn may be affected by legal, political, religious and cultural considerations. Some of the factors involved are discussed below. However, programme planners may decide to test initial acceptance

---

[a] Depot-medroxyprogesterone acetate (DMPA) and cancer: Memorandum from a WHO Meeting. *Bulletin of the World Health Organization*, **64**: 375–382 (1986).

of a new method by conducting a field study. Chapter 9 describes why and how this might be done.

Characteristics of the client

Pregnancy and family planning history. Among women who already have children, their previous experience of pregnancy and delivery may influence their decision whether or not to use contraception for family spacing or limitation. Women who have never been pregnant and who want to postpone childbearing are special cases with respect to the choice of contraceptives. Both groups may, however, need the assurance that there will be no side-effects that could adversely affect future fertility.

Contraceptive history is also important, since the previous experience of users with other contraceptive methods is likely to influence the acceptance of a new method and to lead to certain expectations about it.

Various socioeconomic factors, such as the client's educational level, occupation, and financial status may also affect the acceptance of injectable contraceptives. Other factors to be taken into account include the nature of the client's relationship with her partner, the quality of communication between them, and the degree of joint decision-making.

Characteristics of the provider

Professional commitment. The commitment of the health worker in the community to the use of effective and acceptable contraceptive methods is essential. The attitude of the medical and nursing professions, especially in sectors that may be directly involved, such as obstetrics and gynaecology, paediatrics, community health, maternal and child health, laboratory services and family planning, will affect the acceptance of the method. If national coverage is planned, the cooperation of the private sector, including pharmacists and representatives of the mass media, is useful since adverse opinions or news stories may create anxiety and opposition, both in the private sector and among the public at large.

Attitudes and skills of health workers. The attitudes of staff will influence both method acceptance and

9

continuation of use. Their communication skills—the ability to listen and to respond sympathetically to clients who have questions about any problems that may have arisen—are crucial. They must also, of course, be well versed in the characteristics of other contraceptive methods, since the client will be making a choice.

Characteristics of the method

Clients' perceptions of the method's advantages and disadvantages, including its safety, effectiveness, convenience of use, cost and potential side-effects, will influence their choice. A distinction should be made between the beliefs of the client about the method and those of the provider. It is important that they should be shared and clarified. The effectiveness of injectable contraceptives is discussed on pages 19–20, while safety is considered below.

Safety. Modern hormonal contraceptives are evaluated by means of both animal tests and human studies, and ultimately by long-term surveillance once the preparation is in widespread use.

Epidemiological studies on cancer and the exposure of infants *in utero* are continuing. Those so far conducted on cancer have already been summarized. The published data on potential adverse effects on inadvertently exposed infants have been reassuring. It is, however, important to ensure that long-term monitoring of contraceptive drugs, such as the injectable steroid preparations, is undertaken in all countries in which they are widely used. This will allow any problems not indicated by animal and human studies to be identified and assessed.

All available injectable contraceptives are extremely effective in preventing pregnancy (see page 20). However, they also have a number of adverse effects for some women. The major advantages and disadvantages of these contraceptives are described below. A few important beneficial non-contraceptive side-effects have also been demonstrated and others are being studied.

Advantages and disadvantages. The *advantages* of injectable contraceptives will vary in importance depending on the user, but include the fact that they are highly effective, reversible, and relatively long-lasting. Studies have shown that they can safely be used over a period of several years, and are not dangerous to health, provided that there are no contraindications (see page 66). In some cultures, the use of an injection will be considered an advantage while in others the opposite may be true. A number of conditions may also improve with the use of injectable contraceptives, e.g., iron-deficiency anaemia.

The major *disadvantage* is the probability of irregular bleeding. The rare episodes of heavy bleeding may require professional attention, but no damage to health is caused by other irregularities of bleeding. Another disadvantage is that, once administered, the contraceptive effect lasts until the drug has been fully metabolized by the user; with DMPA, this may occasionally take up to 6 months after the end of the 3-month period of action.

The various advantages, benefits and disadvantages are listed below.

Advantages

- Very high overall use-effectiveness rates, better than for oral contraceptives in some countries.

- No estrogenic side-effects.

- Suitable for lactating women.

- Reversible.

- Trained health workers other than doctors can prescribe and administer them.

- Acceptable in many cultures.

- Independent of coitus.

Non-contraceptive benefits

- Endometriosis can improve.

- Vaginal candidiasis and pelvic inflammatory disease occur less often than, for example, in women who use an IUD.

- Homozygous sickle-cell disease may be ameliorated.

- Iron-deficiency anaemia may be improved.

11

- Pre-existing ovarian cysts and benign breast lumps may recede.

- Production of breast milk is not decreased.

Disadvantages

- Disturbances of the usual bleeding pattern occur in almost all women; this is one of the main reasons for discontinuation. These disturbances may vary from irregular bleeding, spotting, and amenorrhoea to prolonged bleeding, although heavy bleeding is rare.

- Once administered, the effects of the drug last until it has been fully metabolized by the user.

- For some individuals, the administration of an injection is not acceptable.

- Some women gain weight, and complain of feelings of bloatedness and breast tenderness; the weight gain is probably due to increased appetite rather than fluid retention.

- Headaches, mood changes, and loss of libido with use have all been reported. There is no reliable evidence that the incidence of these side-effects is higher than when other forms of contraception are used.

- Return of fertility may be delayed.

Cultural and religious factors

Some features of a particular contraceptive method may give it an advantage in one culture but make it less acceptable in another. For example, the administration of drugs by injection is more acceptable in some cultures than taking drugs by mouth.

The most frequent and significant side-effects reported by women using DMPA and NET-EN are those associated with disturbances of the menstrual cycle, and 25–50% of the women who discontinue the method during the first year of use do so because of these disturbances.

This has important implications for the programme but more importantly for the woman using this method. While she may welcome and benefit from the freedom that a reliable contraceptive method offers, the psychological, social and cultural effects of disruption of bleeding patterns may make the method unacceptable. Programme managers should therefore consider such questions as how a change in bleeding pattern, especially if bleeding is prolonged, will affect a woman's personal relations with her partner, her daily work or her other social, family or religious commitments.

Women should be medically screened (see page 65), if possible examined, and thoroughly counselled by trained personnel before they are given an injectable contraceptive. The sex of the examining person may be important in some cultures, particularly those in which women's bodies may not be exposed to males.

Controversial issues

When a new method is introduced into a family planning programme, managers should consider the attitudes of influential members of the community, such as village and religious leaders, traditional birth attendants or healers and private medical practitioners, as well as of women's organizations and women's health advocacy groups. Their opposition can seriously limit the acceptability of the method.

Managers should therefore be aware of some of the controversial issues and be able to explain the advantages and benefits as well as the disadvantages of injectable contraceptives. A potential user of a contraceptive method must be given the opportunity to discuss the known risks and benefits of the method, together with any other aspects of it that she needs to consider to enable her to make an informed choice.

Other factors

Many women find injectables to be a highly satisfactory contraceptive method. In some family planning programmes where a number of different methods, including injectables, are offered, they are chosen by up to 50% of the women.

The mode of administration partly explains this popularity. In many developing countries people prefer injections because various injected medications have proved to be effective against disease. In Indonesia and Thailand, for example, respect for injections dates back to the successful yaws eradication campaign of the 1950s, which used injections of penicillin.

Injectables are also popular because they require less effort than other methods. Many women prefer a single injection every few months to taking a pill or measuring basal body temperature every day. The injection is not related to the timing of coitus, and women do not have to buy or store supplies. They can discontinue the method simply by not having another injection, whereas IUDs or non-biodegradable implants must be removed by a trained health worker. Also, injectables can be administered outside the home. A woman can maintain her privacy and, if necessary, she can receive an injection without the knowledge of her husband or family.

The quality of the counselling given to a woman or couple about injectables greatly affects satisfaction with the method and continued acceptance of it. A counsellor must first of all be able to listen effectively and to elicit the feelings and thoughts of the client, before providing any advice. The effective counsellor will respect the woman's right to decide, perhaps in consultation with other family members if she wishes, and provide her with sufficient information, clearly and simply presented, so that she can make an informed choice. A decision made in this way is much more likely to be lasting and to foster trust and confidence in the service, so that she will be likely to return for help if needed. (For further information on counselling, see page 55.) In addition, an efficient referral system is important in any injectables programme. With a good referral system, clients can be sure that side-effects will be dealt with and questions answered.

When deciding where to go for services or contraceptives, the factors that individuals and couples take into consideration will include:

- the cost of services;
- their perception of the quality of care provided;

- the anonymity and privacy accorded;
- the dependability of supplies;
- the overall reputation of the source;
- the availability of other needed services at the same place; and
- the distance to alternative sources.

When deciding which method to choose from among a variety of methods offered, clients will take a number of factors into consideration, including:

- the effectiveness of the method;
- the side-effects;
- the safety of the method;
- the cultural and religious acceptability;
- the mode of administration;
- the ease and frequency of administration;
- reversibility;
- the need for close medical supervision;
- the cost of the method.

Factors affecting programmes

Apart from the factors affecting the availability and acceptability of injectable contraceptives discussed in the previous section, programme managers also need to take account of client eligibility, costs and effectiveness when designing and offering services.

Client eligibility

Injectable contraceptives are highly effective in preventing pregnancy for periods of 2 or 3 months, and can be used by all women, including nulliparous ones, provided that no contraindications exist (see page 66). However, service providers should pay special attention to certain groups of women, and to women at certain times in their life.

Post-abortion and postpartum use. Any of the progestogen-only contraceptive methods may be started immediately following abortion, or 6 weeks after childbirth. None of them appears to have any deleterious effect on the quantity of breast milk; in some studies, DMPA use has, in fact, been followed by an increase in the amount of breast milk produced and in the duration of breast-feeding. Infants whose mothers received DMPA while breast-feeding appear to develop normally both physically and mentally. Current studies have followed them as far as 13 years of age.

There is some evidence that a few women may experience episodes of heavy endometrial bleeding if DMPA is started too soon after childbirth. It is therefore advisable to wait for 6 weeks following delivery before this preparation is given.

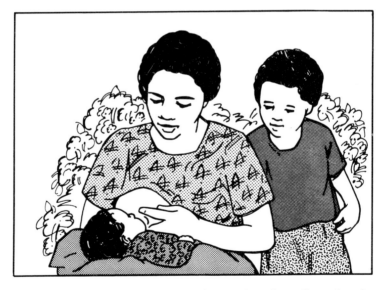

Fig. 2. Injectable contraceptives can be used as from 6 weeks after childbirth.

Women in later reproductive years. A number of difficulties may arise for users of progestogen-only contraceptives in this age group, since it may be difficult to determine the onset of menopause and the concurrent end of any need for further contraception. Problems arise mainly because of the irregular bleeding patterns associated with the methods. On the other hand, the amenorrhoea and irregular menstrual periods that frequently occur in users of progestogen-only contraceptives may be mistaken for signs of the menopause and contraceptive use may be discontinued prematurely. Finally, there is the theoretical concern that irregular bleeding in this age group may be a sign of underlying gynaecological disease. It is very uncommon for this to be the case in long-term users of injectables; however, a woman over 40 years who shows a change in bleeding pattern may need to be investigated for possible cervical disease, including cervical cancer. Endometrial cancer is rare in women who use these contraceptives, and diagnostic curettage to rule out this condition is rarely necessary. This diagnostic procedure should be considered only if the woman is in a high-risk group for the condition and the clinical signs are suspicious.

Adolescents. Concern has occasionally been expressed about the administration of hormonal contraceptives to adolescents (within the first 1 or 2 years after the menarche). The effects of such hormonal use on later sexual development and reproductive function are not fully understood and caution is usually advised if any hormonal method is prescribed within the first 2 years after the menarche. However, if sexually active adolescents are not able to use other methods, the use of hormonal methods should not be regarded as absolutely contraindicated. It is usually felt that the medical, social and psychological consequences of unwanted pregnancy and therapeutic abortion in adolescents outweigh any physiological reservations that currently exist with regard to use of hormonal contraceptives.

It should be noted that, in older adolescents, hormonal contraceptive methods carry a very low risk in terms of metabolic changes and clinical complications and that these methods may have some clear advantages in this age group (such as a significant degree of protection against pelvic inflammatory disease).

Women with pre-existing chronic disease. Many women in this group may face an increased risk of complications if they become pregnant, so that highly effective contraception, such as that provided by hormonal methods, may be particularly desirable. A risk–benefit comparison between the possible hazards of contraception and those of pregnancy should therefore be made. The outcome will be different from that of an analysis of this type in women with no such increased risk of complications. Several of these conditions are discussed on pages 68–69.

Other groups. Other groups of women that may benefit from DMPA and NET-EN use include those who:

- have medical contraindications to other methods;
- are unwilling or unable to use other methods;
- have experienced prior contraceptive failure;
- wish not to have any more children but do not wish to be sterilized;
- lack the continuous motivation necessary with other methods.

Costs

The costs of providing injectable contraceptives through a family planning programme vary widely from one country and type of programme to another. The cost of the injectable product is affected by many factors, including:

- availability of donations or subsidies from external agencies;
- quantity ordered;
- shipping costs.

Product costs alone, however, are not the only determinants of the total cost of contraceptive provision.

The following are some of the other factors that affect overall cost:

- development of informational materials;
- treatment and management of method-related side-effects;
- ease of service; it is generally less expensive to serve urban dwellers, for example, than those living in isolated areas;
- transport, storage, maintenance of premises and equipment;
- staff salaries and training;
- extent to which the existing health care system needs to be modified.

Comparative costs. Contraceptive methods that require regular resupply, e.g., injectables, oral contraceptives and barriers, are likely to be more expensive over time than permanent (sterilization) or long-term methods (IUDs and implants). Of those that do require resupply, injectable contraceptives offer several cost advantages. The initial product cost is relatively low and the contraceptive does not necessarily have to be administered by a physician or nurse.

Calculating cost-effectiveness. Many techniques can be used to determine the cost-effectiveness of different contraceptives. Some are highly sophisticated and precise while others are simpler to use and provide only basic estimates. One practical and simple technique that can be used to provide *general* estimates of the relative costs and cost-effectiveness of contraceptive methods is described in the booklet *Assessing the characteristics and cost-effectiveness of contraceptive methods*, which is available from the Program for Appropriate Technology in Health, (PATH) (see Annex 2).

Effectiveness

The effectiveness of a contraceptive method is usually the most important factor both for the individual or couple

19

trying to choose a method and for the family planning provider involved in counselling them. Potential users need to know how reliable a given method is, while family planning providers need to know how far they can depend on the various methods to prevent pregnancies.

In presenting failure rates for couples in such a way that valid comparisons can be made between methods, it is advisable to present the failure rate both for those who use the method consistently and correctly and that for typical users of the method. Data presented in this way for a number of contraceptive methods are shown in Fig. 3.

Pregnancy rates. The results of clinical trials have shown that both DMPA and NET-EN are highly effective contraceptive agents. Pregnancies due to method failures have been consistently low with the use of 150 mg of DMPA given every 90 days—usually considerably less than 1 pregnancy per 100 woman–years after 12 months of use, and less than the rate for combined oral contraceptives.

The pregnancy rates reported with NET–EN use have varied according to the interval between injections.

In view of the available data, the WHO Task Force on Long-acting Systemic Agents has recommended that injections of NET-EN be scheduled every 60 days, but that injections be permitted up to 14 days before or after the 60-day scheduled visit, that is, between 46 and 74 days after the previous injection. This schedule is designed to maximize protection against conception, while remaining flexible enough to be feasible in a local family planning clinic setting.

Continuation rates. Although multicentre comparative trials have shown that both DMPA and NET-EN are highly effective contraceptives, continuation rates vary markedly between different populations and centres.

Irregularities in vaginal bleeding, such as spotting, prolonged bleeding and, rarely, heavy bleeding, usually account for 10–15% of the discontinuations of both the drugs within the first year of use. An additional 11–12% of women using DMPA discontinue because of amenorrhoea. Discontinuations because of amenorrhoea are less frequent (7–8%) among women using NET-EN. However, in field trials, far greater differences in discontinuations for bleeding irregularities and amenorrhoea can be seen

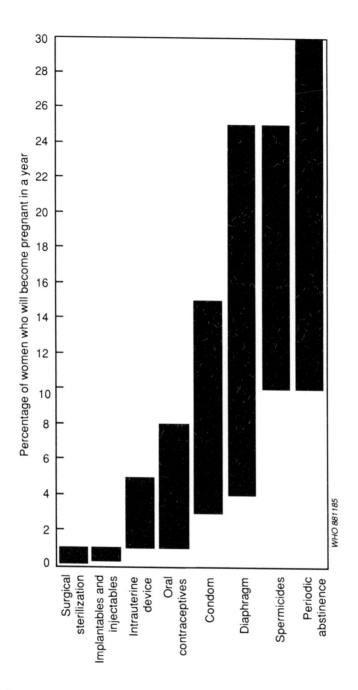

WHO 881185

Fig. 3. Estimated range of failure rates for various contraceptive methods.
Adapted from Mauldin, W. P. & Segal, S. J., *Prevalence of contraceptive use in developing countries*, New York, The Rockefeller Foundation, 1986.

between different populations. It should also be noted that there is a change in the bleeding pattern with length of use of injectable contraceptives: the initial bleeding irregularities become less frequent while the incidence of amenorrhoea increases.

It has been suggested that particularly good counselling could account for low overall discontinuation rates in some centres. It is essential, therefore, to develop appropriate teaching materials to assist family planning clinic personnel in the counselling of subjects in relation to intermenstrual bleeding. (For more information on counselling, see page 55.)

It must be stressed that the effectiveness of a contraceptive does not depend solely on the individual or couple concerned. The managers or administrators of family planning programmes can improve the overall effectiveness and the continued utilization of their clinics by:

- ensuring a dependable flow of supplies;

- maintaining the quality of supplies;

- keeping an adequate stock of materials and instruments for administering the contraceptives;

- making unbiased counselling available;

- providing a reliable follow-up and recall system.

Additional sources of information

ARCHER, E. *Injectable contraceptives. The role of long-acting progestogens in developing countries.* London, Save the Children Fund, 1985.

BENAGIANO, G. & FRASER, I. The Depo-Provera debate. Commentary on the article 'Depo-Provera, a critical analysis'. *Contraception,* **24**(5); 493–528 (1981).

MAULDIN, W. P. & SEGAL, S. J. *Prevalence of contraceptive use in developing countries.* New York, The Rockefeller Foundation, 1986.

Facts about injectable contraceptives: memorandum from a WHO meeting. *Bulletin of the World Health Organization,* **60**(2): 199–210 (1982).

2. Injectables and the health system

Family planning is an important part of the health care of mothers and children because it reduces mortality and morbidity in both. The provision of contraception should therefore be integrated in the health system of the country or community.

Injectable contraceptives are easy to deliver and can be introduced without difficulty into family planning programmes, using existing personnel, facilities, and referral and service delivery channels.

Service delivery channels

In general, to increase coverage and make methods acceptable and readily available to as many people as possible, most programme managers concerned with family planning employ a combination of service delivery strategies within the health care system. In brief, these alternative and complementary approaches include both clinic-based and community-based services.

Clinic-based services

There are two main types of clinic—those that provide family planning as part of an integrated service and those that provide only family planning and/or other reproductive health services.

In the clinics providing integrated services, family planning is provided as part of the maternal and child health and other primary health care services. Such clinics may be part of a national health service or may be paid for and run by nongovernmental organizations, women's groups, etc. In addition, private medical practitioners provide clinic-based family planning services as part of their family health care. In many settings, they form an important group of health care providers who supply injectable contraceptives. Ideally, injectables should be available whenever and wherever other family planning methods are offered in order to avoid disappointing the woman or couple who may wish to use this method.

Clinics are used largely by people living in cities, peri-urban areas and towns. Potentially, the standard of care can be high (side-effects can be treated on the premises and, if the facilities are available, individuals can be screened for anaemia, diabetes, cervical and other forms of cancer, etc.). Also, the cost per user-year tends to be low for all methods because of the large number of people served.

However, in most developing countries, 40–90% of the population live in rural areas and urban slums and do not have reasonable access to clinics. Such people are often not willing to travel long distances for preventive as opposed to curative care.

Services in rural areas can be provided through mobile facilities, usually based in clinics or hospitals. The advantage of this approach is that it takes the service to the community, but operating costs can be very high. The use of mobile facilities for delivery of injectable contra-ceptives should be discouraged unless frequent visits (twice a week) can be made to each community to avoid giving injections to recently pregnant women.

Community-based services

Within communities, local volunteers, usually women (sometimes trained traditional birth attendants), can be recruited to promote family planning and educate their neighbours. As part of their training, community health workers, again including traditional birth attendants, learn to use a check-list to screen for potential complications, to refer women with side-effects associated with the use of a method to a clinic, to take charge of stores, and to keep simple records of the commodities distributed. In some cases, community health workers may also administer injectable contraceptives. However, before a decision is taken to use a non-clinical, non-medical system for the distribution of injectable contraceptives, the following points should be taken into account:

(1) The decision must be taken by the programme authorities and accepted at every level of operation. This sometimes necessitates a revision of the regulations governing health professionals or other legislative changes.

(2) The distribution system must be under the supervision of the national family planning programme.

(3) An important role in the delivery of contraceptive services can be played by nongovernmental organizations if their activities are coordinated by national programmes.

(4) The proper training of all the personnel involved must be guaranteed, and this training should be supervised by the national family planning programme.

(5) Supplies and proper channels for distribution are needed and should be in operation.

(6) The necessary drugs and facilities for the management of bleeding problems should be available (see pages 74–76).

(7) Such a system requires the support of medical facilities to cope with any clinical problems.

The cost to the users of a community-based service is low, while the start-up and recurring costs for the programme are high. The major advantages of this approach are: (1) communities can feel that this is *their* service because of their involvement in it; and (2) the programme can reach large numbers of rural women who might otherwise not use a method of contraception at all.

Follow-up and referral facilities

Fig. 4 illustrates the links between the client, the service delivery channels and the referral facilities. The various components of the system are defined below.

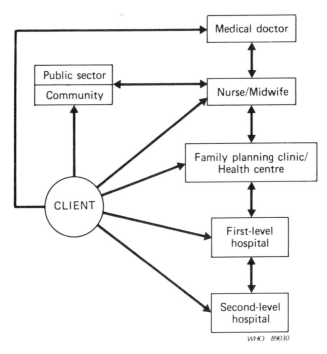

Fig. 4. Links between the client, the service delivery channels and the referral facilities. For explanation, see text.

Client: a potential or continuing user of contraceptive services.

Public sector: a non-clinic facility run by the community dealing with health in general and especially with mother and child welfare, e.g., a village community association or a mothers' association. Paramedical or volunteer health workers at this level must be trained to identify problems and to refer the client to the nearest health centre when serious ones are encountered.

Nurse/midwife: a certified nurse/midwife who has been trained in family planning in general and specifically in injectable contraceptives. He or she is associated with a local doctor and is trained to recognize and refer serious problems early.

Family planning clinic/health centre: a health facility providing basic health care to a community in a certain area.

Hospital I: a district or regional hospital with approximately 50–100 beds, and facilities for dealing with moderately serious problems.

Hospital II: a larger or national hospital with approximately 300 beds and a larger number of specialized personnel.

A client may be given the initial injectable contraceptive, as well as subsequent injections, in any of the above facilities. If she has complaints or side-effects, she must return to the same facility which, if it cannot handle them, will refer her to the nearest higher facility, and so on.

Clients must be given adequate information about possible side-effects and feel comfortable in seeking assistance if they encounter problems.

Supervision of service delivery personnel

Supervisors are responsible for seeing that work in which they themselves are skilled, and which is being carried out by others for whom they are responsible, is being done efficiently and effectively. The task of a supervisor is a demanding one. It requires an understanding that the supervisor's function is that of supporting, guiding and directing the worker, and not simply of giving orders. At the same time, supervisors must develop their ability to carry out the job by dealing with and overcoming all the obstacles placed in their way by others.

The supervisor should be responsible for:

- helping workers plan, implement and evaluate their work;

- providing technical advice;

- handling grievances and disciplinary problems involving workers;

- stimulating and evaluating performance;

- providing continuing education; and

- serving as a link between workers and the central authority responsible for health.

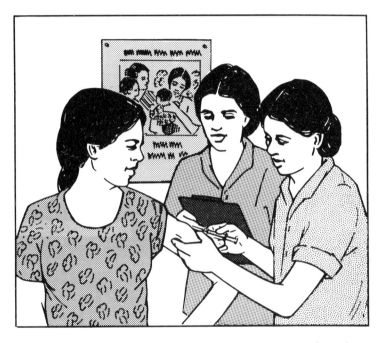

Fig. 5. Appropriate supervision is an important element of service delivery.

Additional source of information

Strengthening of supervisory mechanisms in maternal and child health/FP. Unpublished WHO document FHE/85.5 (1985). Available on request from Maternal and Child Health, World Health Organization, 1211 Geneva 27, Switzerland.

3. Organizing and managing a programme offering injectable contraceptives

This chapter provides the basic information needed by a programme manager to organize and manage an effective family planning programme offering injectable contraceptives.

Check-list for use in planning services

Systematic and thoughtful planning will facilitate the smooth introduction of injectable contraceptives into a family planning programme and will increase the likelihood of success. Table 1 provides a check-list that can be used for planning purposes; the order in which the activities are carried out will depend on local conditions. The table also shows where information on each of the steps can be found in this publication.

Identifying potential obstacles

Potential obstacles to the introduction of injectable contraceptives are:

—political, cultural and religious attitudes and beliefs;

—professional and social attitudes to family planning and to injectable contraceptives in particular;

—relevant local laws, regulations, medical norms, and codes of ethics.

These were discussed in Chapter 1.

Table 1. Check-list for introduction of injectables in a family planning programme

Activity	Sources of information
1. Survey community; identify potential obstacles.	pages 29, 95–98
2. Ensure that national and local legislation and regulations permit use of injectable contraceptives; obtain necessary approvals.	
3. Estimate potential demand and expected caseload.	pages 39–47
4. Arrange programme financing; develop budget.	pages 52–53
5. Identify clinic facilities.	pages 23–27, 31–32
6. Establish essential policies:	
• client-selection criteria;	pages 15–18, 65–67
• counselling and informed consent;	pages 55–58
• medical protocols and medical service standards.	Chapters 5–8
7. Staff the programme:	
• staffing requirements: staffing patterns, types, numbers;	pages 52, 83–86
• recruitment and selection;	
• training;	Chapter 7
• supervision.	pages 27–28
8. Arrange for equipment, supplies, and services:	
• procurement of required equipment, instruments, medicines, and supplies;	pages 37–48
• storage and inventory control;	pages 48–52
• procedures for sterilizing instruments.	pages 32–37
9. Develop a community information, education and communication programme.	Chapter 4
10. Develop and print record forms, informational materials, and documents:	
• medical history/client record form;	Annex 5
• client brochures (e.g., fact sheet);	
11. Establish client-flow system and procedures:	
• reception, intake, registration;	
• record of patient history;	
• client medical assessment and counselling;	
• informed decision;	
• physical examination and medical screening, including laboratory examinations;	Chapters 5 and 6
• referral for further assessment;	
• pretreatment care and preparation;	
• follow-up procedures.	
12. Establish client-referral channels; develop links with other medical, family planning and community institutions and professionals.	pages 26–27

Table 1 (*continued*)

Activity	Sources of information
13. Other: • strategies for marketing, advertising and use of mass media; • financial accounting procedures; • data collection (service statistics) and programme evaluation.	pages 61–62 Chapter 8

A further important obstacle is the effect that injectables can have on a woman's normal menstrual cycle. Managers must be aware of local beliefs and perceptions related to menstruation and be prepared with appropriate information, education and communication materials to help prevent unnecessary fears and alarm.

Facilities

The administration of hormonal injectable contraceptives requires few facilities other than those normally associated with a field clinic. Thus a modest clinic facility for administering injections should contain:

(1) a waiting area for clients;

(2) an examination area where the health worker can counsel clients on the use, effects and side-effects of injectable contraceptives. As part of the counselling process, the potential acceptor should also be given similar information about other available methods of contraception. If possible, a suitable area where physical and gynaecological examinations can be carried out, and an area where the injections can be administered, should also be available;

(3) a cool, secure, well-ventilated storage area for keeping supplies at a temperature of less than 30 °C;

(4) a suitable, secure office area for taking notes and keeping client records;

(5) suitable washing facilities for clients and staff.

The facility should be large enough to accommodate the anticipated number of clients. ("Requirements forecasting", pages 39–44, gives examples showing how monthly/annual demands can be estimated and the size of the facility needed calculated from them.)

Equipment

The administration of injectables does not require a sterile operating room, although hygienic surroundings are important. All instruments used—syringes, needles, gloves and instrument supply tables—must be sterile and pyrogen-free. The quantities of syringes and needles required on an annual basis can be estimated from the forecasts of demand (see pages 37–48). The syringes should be sterile, single-use, disposable devices or sterilizable, reusable instruments. It must be impressed on clinic staff that single-use, sterile, disposable plastic syringes are not designed for recycling and reuse. *These devices are difficult to clean and resterilize and although they may appear*

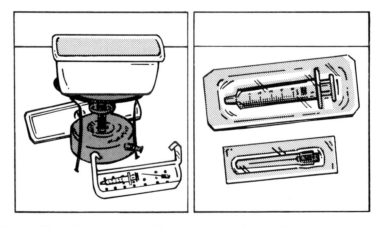

Fig. 6. All syringes and needles used must be sterile.

satisfactory, reuse can be dangerous. Resterilized plastic instruments can fail during use (by snapping or breaking when inserted in the patient), cause serious harm (if leaching of plasticizers into the patient takes place) or be nonsterile and pyrogenic.

Programme managers and staff should be aware that:

- Nonsterile injections can transmit diseases, such as viral hepatitis B and acquired immunodeficiency syndrome (AIDS).

- A sterile needle and a sterile syringe must be used for each injection.

- Changing needles but using the same syringe does not prevent disease transmission.

- Reusable needles and syringes must be taken apart, cleaned and sterilized after each injection.

- Disposable syringes and needles must never be used more than once. If it is impossible to ensure that they will be destroyed after a single injection they should not be used. They must never be sterilized.

- Reusable needles and syringes should be sterilized in a steam sterilizer for 20 minutes at 121 °C.

- If steam sterilization is not available, boiling for 20 minutes in a container with the lid in place will kill nearly all organisms at low altitudes. As the altitude increases so must the boiling time; at high altitude boiling can become ineffective.

- An abscess arising at the place of an injection generally means that an unsterile needle or syringe was used. All abscesses should be investigated immediately and any necessary remedial action taken.

- The public should be made aware of the dangers of unsafe injection practices both within and outside the health services.

The risk of transmitting disease through injections

Injections given with nonsterile syringes or needles increase the risk of transmission of infectious agents, including bacteria, the hepatitis B virus, and the human immunodeficiency virus (HIV) which causes AIDS. However, if strict sterilization practices are observed these risks can be eliminated.

Injectable contraceptives and HIV infection

It should be remembered that injectable contraception is one of the most effective family planning methods and, as such, plays a role in decreasing deaths of women from pregnancy-related causes, improving maternal and child health, decreasing infant mortality through birth-spacing, and reducing the risks associated with illegal abortion.

Since a major cause of HIV infection in children is perinatal transmission from an infected mother, it is essential that women infected with HIV have access to highly effective methods of fertility regulation.

While HIV is readily transmitted through injections given intravenously, the risk from intramuscular injections appears to be low. Moreover, the HIV virus is inactivated at 60 °C and can be eliminated completely with adequate sterilization.

Injection equipment and sterilization

Both reusable and disposable syringes and needles have advantages and disadvantages, as summarized below.

	Advantages	*Disadvantages*
Reusable syringe and needle	● Can be resterilized many times	● Risk of disease transmission if not sterilized properly
	● Unbreakable	● Need for an energy source to carry out sterilization
	● Low cost per injection	
		● Needles can become "barbed"
		● Time required for sterilization

	Advantages	*Disadvantages*
Disposable syringe and needle	• Eliminates transmission risk if properly disposed of after use • No need for sterilization	• Increases transmission risk if not properly disposed of after a single use • Requires a well supervised destruction system • Increases per capita cost of injection

Reusable syringes and needles are likely to be the best option for injectable contraceptives in most developing countries.

The use of reusable syringes and needles calls for good sterilization practices:

- Syringes and needles must be taken apart, thoroughly cleaned and rinsed with water immediately after use, since remaining organic material can harbour infection.

- The dismantled syringes and needles must remain apart so that all surfaces are exposed to the steam or boiling water.

- Simple pressure-cooker-type sterilizers, specially designed for the sterilization of injection equipment, are available through UNICEF. They permit steam sterilization at 121 °C which, if undertaken for 20 minutes, will kill all pathogenic microorganisms, including tetanus spores.

- Boiling injection equipment in water for 20 minutes kills all non-spore forms of organisms known to cause disease in humans, including bacteria, viruses and fungi. However, since the boiling point of water is lower at high altitude, longer periods will be required there. At high altitude, boiling may become inappropriate and steam sterilization must be adopted. At low altitudes if steam sterilization is not available, boiling is an acceptable alternative, but it should be done in a container with the lid closed so that heat and steam stay inside.

Disposable syringes and needles must never be reused. They should be appropriately disposed of and should never be sterilized. Proper sterilization can destroy them. If they fall into the hands of people who are not trained health workers, they may be reused. Disposable syringes and needles are recommended only in circumstances where their destruction after a single use can be assured and where continuous supply can be guaranteed.

Dangerous practices

In many countries, the sterilization of needles and syringes by health workers is not always satisfactory. Some health workers believe they are giving safe injections when in fact they are not. Their mistakes include:

- using the same needle and syringe for more than one injection;
- changing the needle for each injection but using the same syringe;
- not destroying disposable syringes and needles after a single use;
- boiling syringes or needles for too short a time;
- not heating water to boiling point;
- keeping syringes and needles in boiling water throughout the clinic session, taking them from the boiling water as needed and putting them back after use;
- cleaning needles and syringes with alcohol or other disinfectant instead of sterilizing them;
- not cleaning needles and syringes thoroughly before sterilizing them;
- not taking needles and syringes apart before cleaning and sterilizing them;
- storing sterile needles and syringes in a nonsterile container or environment.

Abscesses: an alarm signal

The development of an abscess after an injection generally means that either the injection equipment or the drug was contaminated.

36

The abscesses of primary concern tend to be hot and painful (pyogenic abscesses). They are caused by bacteria, which can be cultured from the abscesses. Often, they occur in a group of women within a short period of time.

Abscesses can be caused through use of a multidose vial that has become contaminated. To avoid such contamination, it is important that:

—any partly used vials are discarded at the end of each clinic session;

—a common needle is not left in the stopper of the vial for withdrawing the drug. Use one needle both to load the syringe and to inject the woman.

Health workers should routinely ask the women receiving injectable contraceptives if any difficulties have been experienced following previous injections, and investigate the cause of any abscesses reported.

Staff who see unsafe injection practices should react to them in the same way they would react to an epidemic of a dangerous disease: immediate remedial action should be taken.

Supplies

For each administration of an injectable contraceptive the following supplies are needed:

- one dose of hormonal injectable contraceptive;

- a suitable skin disinfectant to clean the injection site before and after administration of the contraceptive;

- a sterile syringe and needle. The needle should be 2.5–4 cm in length and 21–23-gauge. The syringe should be graduated to 1.2 ml.

If *disposable* syringes are used, the expiry date on the package should be checked.

If *reusable* syringes are used, it will be necessary to have some means of resterilizing them. This should preferably be done in a steam sterilizer, but if this equipment is not available, reusable instruments can be boiled.

The number of reusable syringes needed in a given situation can be determined as follows. First calculate the time taken to sterilize a full load under the sterilizer's normal operating conditions, and then the number of doses of contraceptive that can typically be administered during this period. For example, if the typical sterilizer cycle takes 120 minutes, and 24 doses (one every 5 minutes) of an injectable contraceptive can be administered in this time, then the facility will require 3×24 sterilizable pieces of equipment (72 syringes, 72 needles). This is because at any one time:

1 set of 24 instruments is being used;

1 set of 24 instruments is being washed and prepared for sterilization; and

1 set of 24 instruments is being sterilized.

Administering an injection is such a simple procedure that mobile health workers can carry a day's supply with them in the field and provide contraceptive injections in remote areas away from an established clinic. If this is done, care should be taken to ensure that the injectable contraceptive is not exposed to temperatures above 30 °C (the normal maximum storage temperature) for periods longer than 1 or 2 days. Additionally, unless manufacturer-supplied, prefilled disposable syringes are used, the syringes for the administration of injections should not be loaded until immediately before use.

Other equipment and instruments

The equipment and instruments required are those normally needed in a comprehensive family planning clinic:

—a scale for measuring weight;

—a blood pressure meter (sphygmomanometer);

—an examining couch;

—instruments for carrying out a gynaecological examination;

—gloves;

—a good light (if natural light is not adequate).

Requirements forecasting

There are two important occasions when it is necessary to forecast the material requirements of family planning programmes—when a new method is introduced and when product demand is monitored.

Introduction of a new method

When a new contraceptive method, such as the use of injectables, is introduced or a change is being planned, the initial and long-term material requirements must be estimated. If the estimates are correct, adequate financing and/or donor assistance can be arranged in advance, sufficient storage space provided, and an overall logistics review carried out to ensure that all levels and components of the delivery system—providers, health workers, motivators, administrative staff, transport, information, storage, etc.—will be able to act in harmony without any one becoming overloaded. Annexes 2 and 3 list the main international sources of assistance for injectable contraceptive programmes and the principal manufacturers of the contraceptives.

Monitoring of demand

Monitoring of demand for injectable contraceptives is essential if undersupply or oversupply is to be quickly corrected. A shift in emphasis can be expected when the programme enters its steady state or equilibrium stage, where the number of new users levels out to a fairly constant percentage of newly eligible women and about the same number of existing users drop out of the programme. During this phase, the task of logistics management is to make fine adjustments to the commodity supply system so as to minimize inventory and transport costs while maintaining availability of product.

Material requirements

Material requirements during start-up, as well as in the later phases of provision of the contraceptive, will depend on the targets set in the overall family planning programme plan. However, independent calculations of requirements can improve the logistics manager's understanding of the factors affecting these requirements.

The following key variables must be known or estimated before meaningful and achievable user targets can be set:

A. Demographic data:

- the number of women of childbearing age, and the age distribution within this group;

- the rate at which this population is expected to increase during the period in which the new contraceptive product is available.

B. Medicosocial data:

- the percentage of eligible women who are not using contraception and who could be expected to accept the injectable method;

- the percentage of eligible women who are now users of other methods and who may switch to the new method;

- the expected discontinuation rate for women who start using injectables.

C. Programme resource data:

- the number of staff available, including motivators/ outreach workers, interviewers, nurses, doctors, clinical support staff and administrators, and their case-handling capacity;

- the geographical distribution of the field workers (caseloads in all parts of the country should be the same);

● the space available for stocking the new contraceptives at both the central and peripheral levels.

Planning for procurement of injectables

When a new contraceptive method is introduced into a family planning programme, programme planners will usually increase the medium-term and long-term targets for fertility control and reapportion the percentages of women using each of the available methods. This re-estimation should take into account the demographic, medicosocial, and programme resource data listed above. For purposes of initial logistics planning, a preliminary estimate can then be made of the equilibrium number of users of the new method once the introductory phase is over. A method of calculating this equilibrium or steady state number of users can be found in Annex 4.

Parameters can easily be calculated for use in making a forecast on the basis of which an initial supply of injectables can be procured and an approximate picture of future needs obtained.

Table 2 shows an example of such a calculation based on the following assumptions:

(1) A three-year start-up phase will attract 300 000 new acceptors per year, subsequently dropping to around 200 000 per year. The rate of population growth of this group is 3% per year.

(2) The discontinuation rate is expected to be 30% of users per year.

(3) The loss of materials due to waste, spoilage or theft is 5% per year.

(4) The dosing frequency is 4 times a year.

Materials management after start-up

Logistics management involves two major tasks after the planning and start-up phases have been completed. In terms of procurement, it is important to make fine adjustments to the system to ensure that sufficient supplies are always on hand at all levels, while at the same time

Table 2. Example of calculation of initial supply of injectables and future needs (all users and doses ×1000)[a]

Item	Year 1	Year 2	Year 3	Year 4	Year 5	Year 6
Number of users carried forward	0	210	357	460	462	468
Number of women joining programme	300	300	300	200	206	212
Number of users discontinuing	90	153	197	198	200	204
Number of users in programme at end of year	210	357	460	462	468	476
Annual number of doses required	840	1428	1840	1848	1872	1904
Inventory losses	42	71	92	92	94	95
Total annual number of doses required	882	1499	1932	1940	1966	1999

[a] For assumptions, see text.

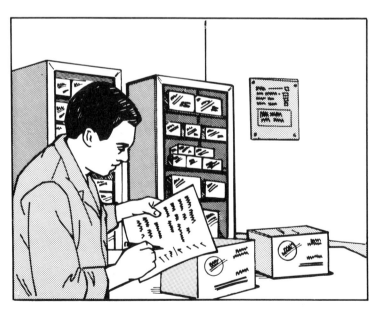

Fig. 7. It is important to ensure that sufficient supplies are on hand at all times.

avoiding oversupply and its attendant high costs. The task
is then that of matching procurement closely to demand
and providing a minimum buffer stock to allow for
unexpected delays, seasonal variations and changes in
demand.

Seasonal variation. One aspect of demand that should be
taken into consideration is seasonal variation. Unless new
supplies are ordered from suppliers only once a year, the
overall efficiency of the logistics process can be improved
by matching orders to the demand forecast for the period
when the supplies are received and distributed. For
example, data from other contraceptive programmes can be
used or, after a year of operation, monthly variations in
acceptance rates or clinic attendance can be correlated with
known causes, as indicated in the example shown in
Table 3.

If the contraceptive reorder interval is 3 months, the
information given in Table 3 could be used to increase or
reduce the size of the order for each quarter by the
percentage shown in parentheses.

Table 3. Example of seasonal variation in attendance at family planning
clinic

Month	Special circumstances	Monthly attendance	Quarterly attendance
January	—	110 000	
February	—	100 000	260 000 (−16%)
March	Festival preparation	50 000	
April	Harvest	75 000	
May	—	120 000	340 000 (+9%)
June	—	145 000	
July	—	180 000	
August	Monsoon	85 000	305 000 (−2%)
September	—	40 000	
October	Planting	55 000	
November	—	160 000	340 000 (+9%)
December	—	125 000	
	Total	1 245 000	
	Average	103 750	311 250

Changes in demand. A further task in logistics management is to keep abreast of, and preferably to anticipate, changes in demand consequent on changes in factors such as discontinuation rates, the dissemination of information, whether favourable or unfavourable, changes in enrolment criteria, cut-backs in motivational programmes, or shortfalls in reaching targets. For this purpose, a management information system is required, which must be properly used by those responsible for logistics management.

Order frequency

The frequency with which orders are placed is determined by the distance from the supplier, the frequency of supply and the speed with which the supplier responds to orders, the dependability of the means of shipment and the warehousing space available to the programme.

Order quantities

Distinct cost advantages and disadvantages are associated with placing large, infrequent orders with the supplier, particularly when the supplier is a manufacturer rather than a donor. The main advantages are the ability to negotiate discounts for such orders, and to economize on the cost of overseas shipping thanks to the savings achieved by qualifying for the use of large containers and for bulk shipping rates. Additional savings resulting from large, infrequent orders are those made in processing the order (fees paid to customs brokers and banks are often the same regardless of the shipment size) and in handling charges incurred at ports and in land transportation. In addition, if the supplier is a donor agency, any problems arising from its inability to respond quickly to frequent small orders are avoided.

Offsetting these substantial savings are the need for very large warehousing facilities (large areas of which will often be left unused as stock levels dwindle), the risk of running out of stock if the shipment is delayed and, in the case of direct purchase, the tying up of greater amounts of foreign currency in large inventories. Large shipments are usually composed of many different batches of the manufacturer's product. In this situation, there is the possibility that some batches may reach their shelf-life expiry date prior to use. Receipt of large shipments also alters normal warehouse routines. When this happens, the risks of incorrect product shipments and other mistakes occurring are increased.

Because of these disadvantages, the placing of large, infrequent orders is not recommended, despite the substantial cost savings to be made.

An acceptable alternative to placing large orders is to negotiate pricing and delivery commitments from suppliers or donors. In the case of commodity purchase, these negotiations are based on a guarantee to purchase a given amount of product over 1 year (or over the programme's life), with the proviso that the purchaser can submit orders at frequent intervals so as to stagger shipment.

Although injectable contraceptives have a shelf-life of over 3 years, placing orders on a quarterly basis is sound practice. When supplies are ordered 4 times a year, the July order, for example, should cover the product requirements for January, February and March of the following year.

Minimum stock levels and order points

Depletion of stock is easily prevented if the significance of two stock levels is always borne in mind: the order point and the minimum stock level.

For practical day-to-day management of contraceptive supplies, it is useful to think of the stock level of any item as a variable which reaches its maximum level when the stock is replenished from the source and then falls as stock is consumed or sent to other places.

The minimum stock level is usually taken as equal to the quantity normally consumed in the period of time between the placing of an order and actual receipt of the supplies. If the manager of the supply system always tries to place orders in time and for the correct amount, the stock should never normally fall below this level. Consequently, the minimum stock level serves as a *buffer stock* which will always be on hand in case of delays in shipment or unanticipated demand.

The order point is the level to which the stock in hand has fallen when an order for new supplies is placed. If this order point is set at twice the minimum stock level, the stock level will continue to fall after the order has been placed but should not be less than the minimum stock level by the time the new supply arrives.

The actual determination of the minimum stock level and order point is left to the discretion of the logistics or warehouse manager. If supply lines are unreliable, the minimum stock level should be increased. When the order point and minimum stock level are calculated for the major warehouse receiving drugs directly from the manufacturer or donor agency, a time schedule should be worked out for the various stages in the order-processing/goods-delivery cycle, as shown in the following example:

	Weeks
Obtain internal management approval for the purchase	2
Obtain foreign currency allocation from central bank (if necessary)	3
Place order with manufacturer or donor and wait for production	14
Manufacturer or donor prepares shipment	2
Freight time (say, air freight)	1
Customs clearance at the port of entry	1
Port clearance and shipment to warehouse	1
Total order time:	24

Some of the items listed above are relevant only to the purchase of supplies as opposed to the receipt of commodities from a donor.

In the above example, the major warehouse will have consumed approximately 6 times the average monthly usage of stock while the order is being processed.

Supply requirements

Pharmaceutical contraceptives by their very nature have particular storage and handling requirements. The quality, purity, shelf-life and efficacy of the drug can all be affected by the way the material is stored and shipped. Therefore, when an order is placed, it is essential to make it clear that the supplies ordered will be accepted and paid for only if the following conditions are satisfied:

(1) All packages, cartons and containers associated with the shipment are clearly marked with the following information:

- the product trade name;

- the product chemical name;

- the number of units contained in the package, carton or container;

- the manufacturer's product batch number;

- the manufacturer's expiry date;

- the number of doses in the package, carton or container.

(2) The minimum acceptable remaining shelf-life of the product when it arrives at the purchaser's warehouse is clearly marked. (This is not the same as the product shelf-life given by the manufacturer. If a manufacturer certifies that the product has a 36-month shelf-life but it has been held in the manufacturer's warehouse for 18 months, its remaining shelf-life will only be 12 months when the 6-month shipment time is taken into account).

(3) The shipment is accompanied by a certificate issued by the exporting country confirming that the drug is registered and permitted to be sold in that country, in conformity with the WHO Certification Scheme on the Quality of Pharmaceutical Products moving in International Commerce.

Although not essential, it is preferable that the shipping cartons are hermetically sealed in clear plastic film. This helps to keep the shipment clean and dry and to keep the various cartons together. Additionally, shrink-wrapping reduces the chance of loss.

The notarization of all documents relating to the shipment by the importing country's consulate before dispatch may minimize delays at the port of entry.

Storage of supplies

The principle of operating any pharmaceutical warehousing system is that the warehouse must be designed and operated in such a way as to minimize any damage to the products while they are stored there.

The above simple statement dictates a whole way of life as far as the design and operation of warehouses are concerned. Injectable contraceptives are relatively stable products but are sensitive to extremes of heat and light. A warehouse for these products must be designed to provide sufficient ventilation to maintain a temperature of 15–30 °C and to protect the products from exposure to direct sunlight. Exposure to unfavourable conditions of heat, humidity and sunlight is sometimes unavoidable, e.g., during transportation, but such exposure should be kept to a minimum. For example, a sealed shipping container should not be allowed to remain outside a warehouse for several days while space is found to store the product. Temperatures inside containers frequently rise to over 50 °C—well above recommended storage temperatures—and this may adversely affect the product.

The warehouse must be large enough to accommodate average monthly usage levels of injectables, as well as other products that have to be stored. If, for example, the warehouse manager has decided that a quarterly order should arrive at the warehouse when the inventory has fallen to the average monthly usage (in this case the minimum stock level is the same as the average monthly usage), the warehouse must be able to accommodate stock levels of 4 times the average monthly usage (the average monthly usage on hand in the warehouse and the newly received quarterly shipment of 3 times the average monthly usage). However, if the quarterly shipment is delayed and arrives shortly before the following one, the warehouse may have to accommodate stock levels as high as 5 or 6 times the average monthly usage. For emergencies such as these, the warehouse must be large enough to store the excess stock or provision must be made for additional storage space elsewhere.

In addition to the space allocated to the pallets carrying the injectables, an approximately equivalent area will be required for movement aisles, areas for receipt of goods and preparation of shipments, and the warehouse staff office and rest-room.

As a precaution against damage by flooding, injectable contraceptives should never be stored directly on floors or against walls. In addition, if this precaution is taken, insect and rodent control programmes and general sanitation activities within the warehouse can be carried out more easily. Ideally, each product batch of stored injectables should be placed on its own pallet (both wooden and plastic pallets are acceptable). When placed on pallets, the batches are easier to move, thus facilitating rearrangement of the stock. Pallets can either be stacked on the floor or on racks or shelving. If space is limited, stacking should be considered only when it is certain that the material on the bottom pallet will not be damaged as a result.

Standard good storage practices developed by the international pharmaceutical community, as described in the booklet, *Management of drug purchasing, storage and distribution* (see p. 54), should be followed.

All products must enter and leave the warehouse in the order in which they are received, i.e., those products received first should also be the first to leave the warehouse. This principle—first in/first out—should ensure that no product in the system exceeds its expiry date (shelf-life) and consequently needs to be destroyed.

The only certain method of ensuring that the principle of first in/first out is put into practice is to use a movement ticket to document all movement of materials into, within and out of the warehouse. A simple but adequate stock control record form for a pharmaceutical warehouse is shown below. This form should be adapted to local needs and languages. In addition to providing an accurate record of the quantities in the warehouse, the record provides essential data on where the products are sent after leaving the warehouse. If a manufacturer needs to recall a product (e.g., because of mislabelling), the record allows all shipments from the warehouse to be easily traced and recalled.

Stock control record   Product lot no. _____

Product name _____   Lot expiry date _____

Manufacturer's name _____   Stores location _____

Date received in stores _____ Zero stock verified by _____.

Movement date	Movement ticket number	Quantity received (in)	Quantity dispatched (out)	Balance (quantity in stock)	Destination of materials

---

Distribution systems

Distribution systems should be designed and implemented in a manner that ensures that the product is shipped between warehouses and from the warehouse to users securely, quickly and with minimum exposure to extremes of temperature and humidity.

When packaged by the manufacturer, the product may be packed in a unit carton. Several unit cartons are then packaged in a shelf carton. The shelf carton is designed to hold a quantity suitable for storage in a cupboard or on a shelf. Typically, the shelf carton may contain 10, 12, 20, 25 or 50 unit cartons, but only rarely more than 100 units. It is strongly recommended that shipments in the distribution chain should not involve breaking up the shelf carton. Shrink-wrapping the shipment (which should be requested in the purchase order) provides protection against humidity and pilfering. When the shelf carton has been shrink-wrapped, both stock control and physical inventory counts are simplified.

Shelf-life and quality control

The product shelf-life indicated by the manufacturer is determined by means of carefully controlled laboratory tests under various conditions. Such laboratory testing guarantees that, if the product is stored under similar or less severe conditions, it will be effective until the expiry date.

A series of quality-control checks should be carried out in the warehouse in order to determine whether the required storage conditions are being met. This is particularly true at the point of receipt of materials. In spite of the best prior planning, products may be exposed to harmful conditions during international or domestic transit.

Incoming quality-control checks should include a thorough examination of the shipment for signs of external contamination since these may be indicative of problems. Water stains on cartons, severe bleaching of printing, tears and rips and animal residues all point to potential product failure. Such occurrences should be noted and, where severe, the shipment refused or examined very carefully.

With all shipments it is usual to select at random some samples for thorough inspection. Some samples of drugs, for instance, may be sent to a laboratory for checking of potency. This may be particularly valuable with a new supplier or a new product type. A new shipment should be carefully segregated on arrival and samples collected in the segregated area. The batch should not be released into the general warehouse area until it is clear that product specifications have been met. If any batches fail the quality-control tests they should be kept separate from other supplies until it is decided either to return the batch to the manufacturer or to destroy the material. Batches that fail any test should never be used in patients.

Quality control also covers the measures taken to ensure that warehousing operations proceed according to standard good storage practices and that any product that has reached its expiry date is destroyed. Products returned by users with complaints should be carefully examined in order to determine the validity of the complaint. Where the complaint is justified, corrective action should be taken to ensure that the fault does not occur again. If users or clinicians complain about specific products, the batches from which these products came should be carefully examined in conjunction with the manufacturer and immediate action taken if the inspection reveals problems.

Record-keeping

There should be no difficulty in adapting client health records for existing family planning methods so as to include important information relevant to the use of injectables. The personal and clinical data that should be recorded for each client are indicated in Chapter 5.

The existing recording and reporting system should be reviewed in order to incorporate the use of injectables in the programme. Provision should also be made for storing confidential health records.

Staffing

The introduction of injectables into an established family planning programme does not necessarily require a change or increase in the type and number of staff. What is important is that existing staff should be fully informed and prepared before the new method is introduced. Administrative, supervisory, medical, nursing and clerical staff should all undergo briefing and, where appropriate, retraining sessions. The skills and training required are outlined in Chapter 7.

Financing

Programme organizers must determine the start-up and recurring costs associated with providing injectable contraceptives through the programme. These will depend on local conditions and particularly on the extent to which the community is involved and helps to support the programme financially.

Most health and family planning facilities will already have the basic equipment and instruments needed for screening and examining clients for injectable contraceptives. Start-up costs may therefore include the costs of:

—public information activities, e.g., through the mass media;

—injectables;

—syringes and needles;

—gloves.

Organizers must plan carefully in order to ensure a steady flow of funds for the programme. Ideally, governments will provide for comprehensive family-planning programmes in their annual budgets. Donor agencies may offer funds, equipment, or technical assistance in starting a programme or to cover the expenses for the first few years. A number of donor agencies are listed in Annex 2. However, organizers should plan from the outset to make the programme self-supporting in the long term. They could consider covering costs by charging fees to clients who can pay. Many programmes have established "sliding fee scales" whereby clients are charged according to their ability to pay or their income. However, clients should not be denied service because of inability to pay.

Characteristics of successful programmes

The criteria for "success" vary from one programme to another, but they are usually related to meeting programme targets combined with a subjective assessment of client satisfaction. In general, "successful" programmes are characterized by:

—an emphasis on quality and client satisfaction;

—activity within the community;

—an efficient and effective system of leadership, supervision and monitoring;

—efficient logistics;

—a good referral system;

—provision of services in a manner convenient to clients.

Additional sources of information

Selection of injection equipment. Unpublished WHO document WHO/UNICEF/EPI.TS.86.2. Available from: Expanded Programme on Immunization, World Health Organization, 1211 Geneva 27, Switzerland.

DÖRNER, G. ET AL. *Management of drug purchasing, storage and distribution: Manual for developing countries*, second revised edition. Available from: International Federation of Pharmaceutical Manufacturers Associations (IFPMA), 67 rue de St Jean, 1201 Geneva, Switzerland.

4. Information, education and communication

The development of a relevant and thorough information, education and communication (IEC) plan is a prerequisite to the successful introduction and continued use of any form of contraception. Health workers must be properly informed about the contraceptive methods that they offer and potential users must be able to make an informed choice from the methods available. Information is given to aid patient choice, and not to persuade, press or induce a person to use a particular method. Furthermore, the decision to refuse a method offered must be based on adequate information just as much as one to accept it. This implies an understanding not only of the effectiveness of that method, but also of the risks involved and the alternative choices possible. To achieve this objective, a variety of interpersonal and public communication skills are essential, and consideration must be given to the training of health personnel and the production of appropriate materials. Clients who have made an informed choice of method are more likely to be satisfied with it and, by talking about their positive experience, become the most effective means of promoting it.

Counselling

Counselling of clients is an essential part of providing contraception and all available methods should be discussed.

In reviewing contraceptive alternatives with clients, health workers should be aware of a number of factors that may be of relevance, depending on the method in question. These will include:

(1) subjective factors associated with the use of any services required, and the time, travel costs, pain or discomfort likely to be experienced;

(2) the accessibility and availability of products that may have to be procured;

(3) the advantages and disadvantages of the method;

(4) reversibility;

(5) the long- or short-term effects.

Once a method has been chosen, counselling should aim to provide the client with a knowledge of the basic facts about the method that has been accepted including, in the case of injectables, accurate information on the following:

(1) how the method works, e.g., how an injection in the arm or buttock can act to prevent pregnancy;

(2) the known contraindications;

(3) the side-effects to expect; in particular, a detailed account must be given of the effect of the injectable on bleeding patterns and the possibility of amenorrhoea;

(4) the management of common side-effects;

(5) the importance for the method's effectiveness of receiving repeat injections on the scheduled dates;

(6) the importance of returning to the provider with questions or complaints that cannot be easily answered or managed by the woman herself;

(7) the importance of regular contact with the health care provider so that the client's health can be monitored;

(8) what will be done during the next visit and why;

(9) the delay (on average 6 months) in return to fertility after ceasing to use an injectable contraceptive.

The importance of fully and clearly spelling out known side-effects to the client cannot be overemphasized. This should be done, however, in such a way as not to alarm the client. It is possible that, if women are told the facts about the method's side-effects, there may be fewer acceptors at first; however, because they have realistic expectations of the method, fewer of them will discontinue at an early stage. All communication with the client must be geared to meet her need for information, and the information must be presented in such a way that she can understand it and feels at ease in asking questions.

The health worker will almost certainly be a very busy individual. Nevertheless, he or she should be encouraged to keep some simple records of the subjective side of the interview; these will be invaluable in evaluating the programme. They might include (in addition to the medical details) some indication of the client's main expressed worry about the method, and any impressions gained on subsequent visits of the *client's* view of any problems. This is likely to provide a clearer understanding of the reasons for discontinuation than the medical records alone.

To encourage the client to express her concerns, simple techniques may be used, such as listening attentively when the client speaks, nodding (or other non-verbal gestures as appropriate) to encourage the client to continue, paraphrasing what the client says to make it more specific but without changing its meaning, reflecting the feelings expressed by the client back to her in a non-judgemental way, asking questions in such a way that the client is not simply reduced to answering "yes" or "no", and ensuring that control of the discussion is not entirely in the hands of the health worker.

In an ideal situation, both partners should be involved in the discussion but this is not always feasible and may not necessarily be desired by the client. As the woman is most likely to be seen initially on her own, she should be encouraged to return, if possible, for a second visit with her partner so that both are fully informed. The initial interview with the woman may, however, give her an opportunity to discuss matters with the health provider that she may be reluctant to raise with her partner present.

A valid decision to use a particular method need not be in writing for legal purposes, because choice is indicated,

not by a signed form, but in freely determined conduct
following adequate discussion. Good practice among literate
patients is to confirm decisions about the choice of contraceptive made during discussions through information sheets
that patients retain. Health workers may then wish to keep
patients' written acknowledgement of receipt. For clients
who have difficulty in reading, health workers should
carefully explain information in simple language with the
help of illustrated brochures and posters. Illustrated
booklets should be given out to these clients.

Printed support materials designed for the specific social,
cultural and educational level of the client can be an
effective means of reinforcing the message conveyed during
counselling.

Training in counselling

Although the techniques of good counselling may seem
self-evident, particular attention must be paid to these
skills in any training programme. (For a discussion of
training, see Chapter 7). As it is more efficient to retain
satisfied clients than to seek new ones, the importance of
counselling should be emphasized to the health worker,
who will most probably be extremely busy and more
accustomed to dealing with medical matters. Staff of the
appropriate level to deal comfortably with clients should be
trained in counselling techniques and properly supervised
by medical personnel.

One of the simplest methods of training in counselling is
the use of "role-playing", in which health workers take
turns at playing the role of client. This can be supplemented by "modelling" of good counselling techniques.

Other audiences for the IEC programme

While contraceptive users are the major target for IEC
activities, there are also other audiences for whom
information about injectables is of crucial importance
because of the role that they may play in the acceptance
of a contraceptive method or, alternatively, in sabotaging

its acceptability and availability. These other audiences may include the following:

- the general public;
- health decision-makers;
- contraceptive providers and other health care providers, especially general practitioners;
- field-workers in family planning or health care;
- specialized groups, including both governmental and nongovernmental agencies, concerned with health, education, religion, social welfare and social policies.

Provision of IEC

Planning an IEC programme

The way can be paved for the introduction of injectables in a community by means of a wide variety of methods, the choice being determined to a large extent by:

- the kind of communication channels that are available and accessible; and
- prevailing beliefs about the method, particularly if it has been the subject of adverse publicity. Information on the controversies associated with injectable contraceptives has been given on pages 4–8.

When any kind of campaign to promote injectable contraceptives is conducted, a number of general factors need to be borne in mind, including the following:

- injectables are not appropriate for all women, so that they should not be oversold;
- those who are developing the IEC programme should be aware of local sensitivities, including cultural or religious taboos;
- groups that are opposed to the use of injectables are likely to be sincere in their beliefs and must be treated with respect;

- the goals of the IEC programme should be established during the planning stage and understood by all those associated with it.

Assessment of information needs

It is absolutely essential for the messages conveyed in an IEC programme to be based on the information needs of the identified target audiences. Thus potential users have information needs that differ from those of health care decision-makers and from those of the general public. In addition, the degree of detail of the message will vary, depending on the needs of the audience. Health workers who will be providing injectables will need to have a much greater knowledge of the method than the general public.

Group discussion with members of the target audience is an important means of information on educational needs. Small group discussions are particularly successful for this purpose. These are conducted as open-ended conversations,

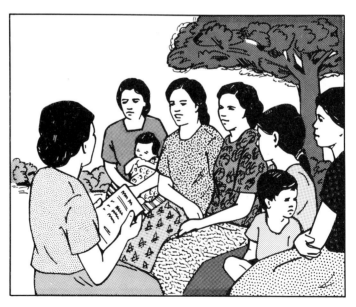

Fig. 8. Group discussion is an important means of providing information and of obtaining feedback on family planning services.

usually 1–2 hours in length, in which all participants are encouraged to interact with one another, to comment on various topics, to ask questions of one another, and to respond to others' comments.

As noted above, discussions with key figures in each of the target groups will be invaluable in preparing the way for any promotional activities. In addition to helping to develop the communication messages, meetings with members of the target audience can help to reduce potential problems in the future. Asking people for their views, and for suggestions as to how the method may best be promoted, includes them in the decision-making process; they may later be instrumental in persuading others to use it. In the course of this "research", sound information can be provided to these key individuals, thereby avoiding the subsequent dissemination of misinformation.

Once the messages for the IEC campaign have been developed they should be pretested with members of the target audience before being finalized.

Channels of communication

Numerous methods of disseminating information can be used in an IEC programme, but the choice will depend on what is available in the country concerned. The channels of communication that can be used include the following:

- the mass media, including radio, television, cinema, newspapers and, increasingly, videos;

- printed materials developed specifically for injectables and relevant to local conditions, including books, leaflets, posters, circulars, comic books, flip charts, etc.;

- personal communication by means of public speakers, group discussions and seminars, theatre, popular music, etc.

These can be used in a wide variety of imaginative ways, some of which must be paid for, e.g., advertisements or the making of a video. Many others, however, are free, such as presentations (e.g., on radio programmes, or in community groups) by interested individuals who are already celebrities and who may be willing to lend their names or their talents, letters to newspapers or magazines, radio phone-in programmes, etc.

The advantage in using any public channel of communication is that large numbers of people can be reached. However, there is also a risk of misinformation or misunderstanding, particularly when the communicators are not sufficiently familiar with the subject matter or able to deal adequately with difficult questions. The individuals who are to take part in such activities must be carefully selected and trained.

The publication *Print materials for non-readers: experiences in family planning and health* discusses many of the issues involved in the development of IEC print materials and provides a methodology for this purpose. It is available from PATH, 4 Nickerson Street, Seattle, WA 98109, USA.

Special groups

Two groups of particular importance for the IEC process are women's organizations and other nongovernmental organizations and traditional midwives and healers; these are discussed in some detail below.

Women's organizations

Women's organizations have demonstrated great concern for women's right to make their own decisions concerning reproduction and for the provision of high-quality care through the service delivery system. In many countries, these organizations can play an important role in communicating with potential acceptors of contraceptives.

It is therefore important to ensure that women's organizations are well informed about methods of contraception by inviting representatives to learn about the contraceptive services available. This is particularly important when new methods are introduced, as there is a tendency for misinformation to generate fears that the methods will be harmful to women and that women are being experimented on. Women's organizations should have an opportunity to discuss both the health benefits and risks of all available methods, and the relevant scientific information should be clearly explained. Family planning workers will benefit also from a dialogue with those with concerns regarding injectable contraceptives. Negative attitudes, particularly those based on misinformation, can jeopardize a good family planning programme and therefore merit full discussion.

Women's organizations, such as mothers' clubs, especially at local and village level, usually hold regular meetings. The members often keep in close contact with one another. Speakers are sometimes invited to address such women's groups on a wide range of subjects, and family planning could be among the subjects discussed. A knowledgeable and understanding speaker can do much to inform about both family planning and the different methods of contraception. Discussions are useful as a means of overcoming any fears and anxieties that individuals or groups might have regarding planning in general, or injectables in particular. Leaflets and other materials produced by women's organizations could carry family planning messages stressing the health benefits of the various methods.

Traditional midwives and healers

In many societies, traditional midwives and healers not only attend women during childbirth but also provide health care to the family, and may be the only available source of assistance on health-related matters. These individuals should be identified and given the necessary information on family planning. Their cooperation and understanding are essential to the success of the family planning programme.

Women are often receptive to family planning information in the immediate postpartum period. The traditional midwife is in contact with these women and can promote the use of contraception, as long as she herself realizes the benefits of family planning and the advantages of the different methods.

Because acting as a birth attendant is often a paid function of traditional midwives, the possibility of giving these women some sort of financial reward for their

63

participation in the family planning programme should be considered.

Summary

The provision of counselling and information in the promotion of injectables must, in common with the introduction of any method of health promotion, satisfy a number of requirements. Those responsible must be sensitive to the client's perceptions and the attitudes and beliefs of those who surround them. Soundness of information, a respect for other people's opinions (particularly if they differ from one's own) and skill in communicating, which above all implies the capacity to listen, are fundamental to success in the use of the method, as with any other.

Advance programming is necessary in order to be prepared for the rumours of side-effects, etc. which sometimes circulate about contraceptive methods. A decision needs to be made as to the best way to counter them, usually by means of sound information provided to the general population.

5. Pretreatment care and administration

All women considering using long-acting hormonal contraceptives must be adequately screened in order to assess their suitability and to determine which of the methods is most appropriate for them.

Since injectable contraceptives are effective for varying periods of time, it is important to know whether the woman wishes to use the method for spacing or for limiting her family. DMPA, which is given every 3 months, inhibits ovulation for a varying period of time following cessation of use. A large study conducted in Thailand showed that, on average, women became pregnant 5.5 months after the presumed end of contraceptive protection with DMPA. NET-EN is given every two months and, while there are no conclusive data, it might be expected that fertility would return more quickly than after DMPA use.

Medical screening

The purpose of medical screening is to determine:

(*a*) the indications for use;

(*b*) whether any contraindications exist;

(*c*) whether there are any special problems that require medical assessment.

Screening usually involves taking a personal and medical history and carrying out a physical examination. Other tests may also be necessary. All findings and important information must be recorded, usually on a client record form.

Indications for use

DMPA and NET-EN are particularly suitable for women who find other methods of contraception unsuitable or unacceptable, e.g., women who are unreliable pill takers. As already pointed out (page 3), women who require maximum protection following rubella immunization, or who are partners of men undergoing vasectomy, or who are awaiting sterilization are also appropriate potential users of injectables.

There are other special groups of users for whom these methods offer a number of advantages as compared with others (see pages 10–11).

Contraindications to use

The contraindications to the use of all forms of long-acting hormonal contraception are as follows:

—pre-existing or suspected pregnancy;

—suspected or undiagnosed breast pathology;

—suspected genital tract neoplasia;

—active viral hepatitis A;

—coagulation or lipid disorders;

—cardiovascular disorders;

—undiagnosed abnormal uterine bleeding.

The contraindications to the use specifically of DMPA and NET-EN are:

—early postpartum administration: delaying the first administration until the sixth week postpartum has been found to reduce the likelihood of heavy or prolonged bleeding and any effect of the drug on the infant via the breast milk is minimized;

—a planned pregnancy in the near future.

So far, there has been no demonstrated interaction between injectable contraceptives and other drugs. Thus, it is likely that DMPA and NET-EN can be used by women being treated with antibiotics or enzyme-inducing drugs such as rifampicin.

Medical history, physical examination and other investigations

A good medical history followed, where possible, by a physical examination is necessary for women who are starting to use DMPA or NET-EN. Where possible, these should be repeated annually, for as long as the woman continues to use injectable contraceptives. They should provide at least the information required to identify those who have contraindications to use or who present special problems that require medical assessment (see page 68).

The medical history should include:

—the date of birth;

—the menstrual history (regularity and length of menstrual flow, occurrence of abnormal bleeding, date of first day of last menstrual period);

—the obstetrical history (parity, abortions, miscarriages, date of last delivery, lactational status, gestational diabetes);

—the medical history (jaundice, other liver disease, cardiovascular disease, blood clotting disorders, diabetes).

The physical examination could include:

—measurement of weight;

—measurement of blood pressure;

—examination of the breasts;

—pelvic examination.

When local circumstances permit, the above may be supplemented by:

—examination of the urine for the presence of sugar;

—a cervical smear;

—a haemoglobin estimation.

Auxiliary workers have been successfully trained to screen potential users and to prescribe and administer injectables.

The health worker should consider the following questions when taking a history:

- Is this type of method or delivery system suitable for this woman or couple?

- Are there any contraindications?

- What are the advantages of this method to this woman or couple?

- Is a medical assessment indicated?

Special problems requiring medical assessment

Most women with pre-existing chronic disease or an undiagnosed condition should have this evaluated before starting hormonal contraception. Thus the following conditions call for medical assessment:

An undiagnosed breast lump. Hormonal treatment may cause such lumps to grow. In addition, the lump should be tested to determine whether it is malignant.

Cardiovascular disease such as hypertension, myocardial infarction, cerebral haemorrhage or thrombosis, or other arterial thrombosis. It is thought that progestogens may play a combined role with estrogens in causing vascular damage in certain women with other high-risk factors for cardiovascular disease, but less likely that such vascular damage will occur with progestogens alone, especially in low dosage.

Previous venous thrombosis. The risk of this condition has been closely linked with estrogen administration, and it is not thought to be a contraindication to the use of progestogens alone. Some authorities, in fact, recommend progestogen-only methods as the contraceptive of choice in these women.

Congenital hyperlipidaemia. Many women with this condition have an increased risk of cardiovascular disease which may theoretically be increased by progestogen use. However, no clinical evidence of this increased risk has been found.

Diabetes mellitus or *history of gestational diabetes.* There is a very small risk of exacerbation with high-dose progestogens, and a theoretical risk of increasing the possibility of cardiovascular disease associated with this condition.

Cigarette smoking. This is known to cause an increase in the incidence of many diseases. Adverse interactions with combined oral contraceptives have been demonstrated, especially in older women, in the causation of several potentially serious cardiovascular diseases. The underlying mechanisms are unclear. It is not known whether they may also apply to progestogen-only methods.

Sickle-cell disease. There may actually be a decrease in the frequency and severity of sickling crisis during DMPA use. However, the condition should always be evaluated first.

A risk of benign liver tumours has been found with combined oral contraceptives but has not been demonstrated for DMPA and NET-EN. Studies on this are continuing.

Check-lists

Check-lists have been developed to assist health workers in identifying women who need medical assessment. They are not an alternative to a full history and physical examination when and where resources permit, but are mainly intended to be used in situations where no doctor is available.

69

A check-list should be drawn up in such a way that conditions which are contraindications to the use of the method can be recognized or the need to refer to a higher level of health care for the management of the patient and a decision as to the method of contraception to be used can be identified.

A sample check-list for use by non-physicians is given below.

		YES	NO
1.	Is the client's period overdue, or is there any possibility that she may be pregnant?	☐	☐
2.	Is the client currently breast-feeding?	☐	☐
3.	Is the client using any drug prophylactically on a long-term basis?	☐	☐
4.	Does the client have diabetes?	☐	☐
5.	Has the client ever had thromboembolic disease, stroke or other cardiovascular disease?	☐	☐
6.	Does the client have or suspect any kind of cancer?	☐	☐
7.	Has the client ever noticed a lump in her breast or any abnormal discharge from the nipples?	☐	☐
8.	Has the client ever had fits, incapacitating headaches, loss of consciousness or paralysis?	☐	☐
9.	Has the client ever had any severe chest pain or shortness of breath after moderate exertion?	☐	☐
10.	During the past 6 months, or during any of her pregnancies, has the client had any illness that caused her eyes and skin to turn yellow, and her urine to turn brown?	☐	☐

If the replies to all these questions are in the negative, the woman may be given an injectable contraceptive.

One positive response does not necessarily mean that injectables are contraindicated, but the potential user should be referred for medical assessment before the preparation is administered.

Recording of information

All the information obtained from each individual should be accurately recorded, usually in a separate record specially prepared for each user or couple.

The health record should be regularly updated to include results of tests or other investigations, a record of each visit, the advice and/or treatment given and any change to the status of the user or couple.

Administration

The importance of adequate counselling before administration cannot be overemphasized. Failure to provide such counselling accounts for much of the adverse publicity about injectables and may cause the user to discontinue the method prematurely (see Chapter 4).

Selection of type of method

Both DMPA and NET-EN are highly effective methods of contraception, with similar side-effects and contraindications. However, since a few differences have been observed between the two steroids, there are situations in which one may be more appropriate as a contraceptive method than the other. The main differences are as follows:

71

- DMPA is given less frequently, namely 4 times a year as compared with 6 times a year for NET-EN.

- DMPA is slightly more effective as a contraceptive.

- There is anecdotal evidence that injection of DMPA is less uncomfortable.

Timing of initial administration

The initial injection of DMPA or NET-EN should be given *during the first 5 days of the menstrual period.* The timing of the initial injection is very important if administration of the contraceptive hormone during early and still undiagnosed pregnancy is to be avoided.

An injectable can be given immediately after an abortion but should be delayed for 6 weeks after childbirth. This reduces the likelihood of prolonged bleeding after administration.

In women who have been taking combined oral contraceptives, injectables should be administered during the days of bleeding immediately after the pill is stopped. In users of minipills (low-dose progestogen-only pills), they should be administered on days 1–5 of the menses. If it is uncertain whether or not the woman is pregnant, steps must be taken to rule out pregnancy before injectables are used.

Before injectables are administered, the woman should, wherever possible, undergo full medical screening and a physical and gynaecological examination, together with any other investigations that might be indicated (see pages 67–71).

The injection procedure

A single sterile needle and a single sterile syringe should be used for each injection. In the few developing countries where disposable needles and syringes are already in wide-spread use, and where they are actually being destroyed after having been used once, the adoption of a policy of using disposable needles and syringes should be considered.

Where the costs and logistics of maintaining supplies are a constraint, reusable needles and syringes may be used.

They should preferably be steam-sterilized after use, but where this is not possible, boiling is an acceptable alternative. Supplies of reusable needles and syringes and sterilizers should be sufficient to ensure that clinic operations are not held up while instruments are sterilized. (See pages 32–38 for further information on syringes.)

Injectables should be administered by deep intramuscular injection into the deltoid or gluteal muscle. Both DMPA and NET-EN may be given with the woman lying down or standing, depending on her preference. If the injection is given in the buttocks, the clinic staff must take account of the woman's need for privacy.

The dose of DMPA for a 3-monthly regime is 150 mg. Vials can contain 1, 3, 5 or 10 ml of a solution containing either 50 mg or 150 mg of drug per ml. The vial should be well shaken before the syringe is charged. It should then be checked to ensure that it contains the correct dosage. When the woman is comfortable, the injection site should be wiped with a disinfectant solution or spirit and the injection given deep into the muscle.

For NET-EN the dose is 200 mg for a 60-day regime. The drug is formulated as a viscous, oily solution which needs special care both when it is aspirated into the syringe and during injection to ensure that all the material is injected and that no leakage occurs around the needle or the barrel. If the vial has been stored at low temperature, it is advisable to warm it to body temperature before giving the injection. Each vial contains 1 ml of a 200 mg/ml solution.

The injection site should not be massaged as this may accelerate the absorption rate of the steroid.

Additional sources of information

Selection of injection equipment. Unpublished WHO document. WHO/UNICEF/EPI.TS.86.2.

How to boil syringes and needles properly. Unpublished WHO/UNICEF document, 1987.

Both these documents are available on request from Expanded Programme on Immunization, World Health Organization, 1211 Geneva 27, Switzerland.

6. Post-administration care

Post-injection advice and care

Immediate side-effects following the administration of an injectable contraceptive have not been reported. The woman should be advised not to massage the site of injection. An anaphylactic reaction to the vehicle used with DMPA has been reported in a very small number of cases. All the reactions, however, were traced to a specific batch of the vehicle in which the steroid was formulated; such reactions are thus highly unlikely to occur.

Counselling does not end once the drug has been administered, since the woman will need to know when and where the next dose will be given; the importance of keeping that appointment should be stressed. This information should be recorded according to the existing practice of the centre and a reminder given to the woman.

Special problems and their management

Changes in pattern of bleeding

A majority of women who receive either DMPA or NET-EN will experience a change in the pattern of their menstrual cycle. Adequate counselling on the anticipated side-effects when contraceptive use is started is essential in order to avoid unnecessary concern on the part of the woman. A woman who has been informed of the possible side-effects and their probable importance to her health will be both less alarmed and better able to judge when she should consult her physician or health worker. The importance of side-effects should not be minimized, however, and she should be instructed to consult her physician or health worker if she experiences prolonged or heavy bleeding.

Every woman who reports prolonged or heavy bleeding should be evaluated for anaemia. It should be emphasized that heavy bleeding is rare and prolonged bleeding is usually scanty and not a threat to health. If a woman is found to have iron-deficiency anaemia, she should receive appropriate oral iron therapy, e.g., ferrous sulfate.

Many clinicians administer estrogen preparations as treatment for bleeding disorders associated with injectable progestogen contraceptives. However, the benefits of this treatment are uncertain. WHO is currently undertaking a multicentre trial to assess the therapeutic effectiveness of two estrogen preparations in prolonged bleeding in women using DMPA.

The approach taken in the treatment of bleeding disorders in clinical trials of both DMPA and NET-EN is

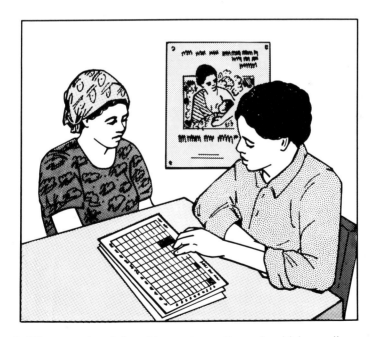

Fig. 9. Women using injectable contraceptives should be well informed about the possibility of bleeding disturbances.

as follows. If the bleeding is heavy or prolonged, the woman should first be examined to exclude a gynaecological cause. One possibility would then be to give the next dose early, but not earlier than 4 weeks after the previous dose. A woman experiencing moderate and prolonged or heavy bleeding due to the steroid could be given 30–50 μg of ethinylestradiol daily for 14–21 days if estrogen is not contraindicated. An alternative is a single 21-day course of a monophasic combined oral contraceptive. If this therapy is ineffective, or if the woman initially presents with very heavy bleeding, she should be given 5 mg of estradiol cipionate or valerate intramuscularly; this dose should be repeated once if the bleeding does not stop or decrease markedly within 24 hours. Additional medical advice may be indicated at this stage. If, after the administration of 10 mg of estradiol cipionate or valerate intramuscularly, the bleeding continues, the woman should be referred for possible dilatation and curettage. A test should be made for anaemia and iron therapy given, if indicated.

Many women can accept bleeding irregularities provided that they are well informed about the underlying causes and are assured that bleeding is neither a sign nor a cause of disease.

Bleeding disturbances are more easily accepted among women who are both highly motivated to use the method and well informed about it and its side-effects.

Amenorrhoea

The likelihood of amenorrhoea increases with increasing use of both DMPA and NET-EN, but women using NET-EN are less likely to experience it than those using DMPA. Prolonged amenorrhoea can lead to anxiety over the possibility of an unintended pregnancy, and this should be eliminated as a cause. If women have been forewarned, they are less likely to be alarmed. Occasionally, a woman may not accept prolonged amenorrhoea and may ask for a "period" to be induced. A single 21-day course of a combined oral contraceptive containing 50 μg of an estrogen may be given if estrogens are not contraindicated.

Conception after discontinuing use

Following discontinuation of DMPA, most women experience a delay in the return of ovulation; this delay varies considerably in length. Thus, women who attempt to become pregnant after discontinuing DMPA will probably have to wait at least several months before conceiving. The average time between the last injection and conception is about 9 months, including the 3 months during which the injection is effective; more than 90% of women become pregnant within 2 years of discontinuing DMPA.

The small amount of information available on conception following discontinuation of NET-EN suggests that the average delay is less than that following discontinuation of DMPA. Women who experience amenorrhoea while using NET-EN appear to take longer to conceive after discontinuation than those who continue to have menstrual periods.

There is no evidence of an increase in the risk of permanent sterility after the use of any injectable contraceptive (see page 79 on return of fertility).

Other side-effects

As mentioned previously, a small weight gain (mean of 1 kg per annum) is reported in nearly all women using injectable contraceptives; this is most probably due to increased appetite rather than fluid retention. Mood changes, loss of libido and headaches have also been reported, but, as pointed out earlier, there is no reliable evidence that the incidence of these side-effects is any higher than when other forms of hormonal contraception are used.

The cardiovascular effects associated with the use of estrogen-containing oral contraceptives have not been found with injectable progestogen-only contraceptives. There appear to be no significant changes in blood coagulation or in the incidence of thromboembolic disease. Effects on blood pressure are minimal; slight decreases have been found in a number of studies.

Possible long-term side-effects

Injectable contraceptives have been used for more than 15 years and clinical evidence thus far has shown no additional and possibly even fewer adverse effects than those found with other hormonal methods of contraception. Nevertheless, postmarketing surveillance of long-term side-effects is continuing in many countries, and is to be encouraged in those not undertaking such activity.

When used responsibly, injectable contraceptives do not appear to impair and may even improve the general health status of women. Their widespread use is likely to produce a substantial reduction in maternal and infant mortality and an improvement in the health of mothers and children.

Possible effects on metabolism

Oral hormonal contraceptives have been associated with effects on a variety of metabolic functions, as shown by changes in coagulation and fibrinolytic factors, platelet function, carbohydrate and lipid metabolism and liver, renal and thyroid function. In most instances, these effects have been considered to be a consequence of the estrogen component. This has been borne out by observations with DMPA, which have shown little or no change in the functions mentioned above except for minor alterations in carbohydrate and lipid metabolism. Few data have been published on the metabolic effects of NET-EN, but its effect on most metabolic functions appears to be similar to that of DMPA.

Risk of carcinogenesis

Until recently, no adequate studies of the effects of DMPA on cancer incidence had been carried out. The previously published data on cancers of the endometrium, ovary, breast and cervix did not demonstrate any increased risk associated with DMPA but, because of methodological limitations, these data provided only limited reassurance. No information is available for NET-EN. In response to requests by Member States and by the scientific community, WHO embarked on a review of all available data on injectable contraceptives and also analysed the data from a WHO multinational collaborative case–control study on neoplasia and steroid contraceptives.

A special meeting was convened by WHO in September 1985 to review both the published and unpublished epidemiological data on the subject. The meeting found that the data from the WHO study did not indicate an increased risk of cancer of the breast, endometrium, ovary or liver in women using DMPA. It is expected that further data will confirm that, like the oral contraceptives, DMPA protects against the development of endometrial and ovarian cancer.[a]

WHO is continuing to monitor the relationship between steroid contraceptives (including DMPA and NET-EN) and the risk of selected neoplasms, including carcinoma of the breast, cervix, endometrium, ovary and hepatobiliary system.

It should be considered as good public health practice to make screening for cervical cancer available to acceptors of steroid contraceptives.

Return of fertility

The presence of MPA in the circulation (following cessation of DMPA use) appears to continue to inhibit ovulation for a varying period of time. As already mentioned, a large study in Thailand showed that women discontinuing DMPA use became pregnant some 5.5 months (on average) after the presumed end of contraceptive protection. The delay in other ethnic groups has not been adequately studied.

The average delay in conceiving was somewhat less for users of IUDs and oral contraceptives, but at 1 year after discontinuation the proportion who had not yet conceived was similar for DMPA and IUD users. At 2 years, more than 90% of previous DMPA users had become pregnant.

---

[a] Depot-medroxyprogesterone acetate (DMPA) and cancer: Memorandum from a WHO meeting. *Bulletin of the World Health Organization*, **64**(3): 375–382 (1986).

Effect on progeny

In utero exposure. No systematic follow-up studies of the health and development of large numbers of infants exposed *in utero* to DMPA or NET-EN have been carried out. When given after pregnancy has begun, DMPA does not appear to increase the risk of spontaneous abortion or stillbirth. No adverse effects were seen on the intellectual development of teenagers who had been exposed *in utero*. Two studies on the sexual behaviour of a very small number of adolescent boys and girls exposed to DMPA *in utero* showed no adverse effects. No studies have been conducted to examine the outcome of pregnancy after exposure to NET-EN.

Exposure of infants via breast milk. Provision of appropriate contraception for breast-feeding mothers is important, especially in developing countries, because the baby's health is dependent on an adequate supply of mother's milk. Thus, DMPA and NET-EN are particularly useful for this special group of women.

Unlike oral contraceptives, which contain both estrogen and progestogen, DMPA does not appear to have any deleterious effects on the quantity or nutritive value of breast milk. In fact, some studies have suggested that there is an increase in the quantity of breast milk with DMPA use.

Both DMPA and NET-EN are secreted in very small amounts in breast milk but no ill effects have so far been found in children who have been exposed to DMPA in this way and are currently being followed up (some of whom are in their early teens). There is also no observed effect of DMPA on adrenal and reproductive hormones during the neonatal period. No equivalent studies have been undertaken with NET-EN.

Follow-up

Regular follow-up of users provides an important opportunity both for assessing any problems and for administering the next injection. It is not always necessary for users to be followed up at a health post or clinic, provided that the visiting local health worker has the necessary instruments and materials. New information must be recorded and entered into the user's personal health record.

Women should be questioned about:

—any problems experienced since the last dose/ appointment;

—the bleeding pattern and date of the last menstrual period.

A follow-up examination should include:

—measurement of weight;

—measurement of blood pressure;

—pelvic and breast examination (annually if possible);

—cervical smear.

It is not essential for women to be seen by a physician at every follow-up visit, but auxiliary staff must be able to recognize cases that need medical assessment, and know how to deal with minor problems.

If periodic evaluation does not reveal any adverse effects, the medication may be continued for as long as desired. In healthy young women the associated risks are minimal.

In women over 40 years of age, a physician should assess general health status before use of an injectable is started or continued. It should be noted that the use of any hormonal contraceptive can mask the onset of the menopause.

Women who are late for their next injection must be reassessed for the possibility of pregnancy and other contraindications. If a woman has been amenorrhoeic and is *not* pregnant the next dose may be given, but it must be strongly emphasized to her that it is extremely important that the next dose be given on time.

It is important to try and find out why women are late for follow-up or fail to attend. The reasons why they may do so include:

● unacceptable side-effects;

- disapproval of husband or other family members;
- failure to remember or understand instructions;
- distance from clinic/health post too great;
- dislike or fear of health personnel;
- cost of travel or method too high;
- adverse reports from friends or relations.

These should be dealt with sympathetically and possible solutions should be explored.

Indications for discontinuation

The medical and non-medical indications for discontinuation of use of injectable contraceptives are discussed below.

Medical indications. If any contraindications to use appear, further injections of the drug should not be given. Similarly, if any of the special problems requiring medical assessment develop, the advice of trained medical personnel should be sought before further injections are given.

Non-medical indications. Any personal reasons for discontinuing the method should be respected and accepted and other methods of contraception made available.

7. Training

Objective

The objective of training is to ensure that the trainee possesses the necessary knowledge and skills to:

—provide comprehensive assessment, counselling and education relevant to injectable contraceptives;

—initiate and manage treatment of clients who choose injectables.

Subjects covered

Two broad categories of personnel, namely medical, nursing, and paramedical staff, and lay workers, may require training in providing injectable contraceptives and in supporting a programme that provides injectables.

Medical, nursing and paramedical staff

Members of this group may be responsible for prescribing injectables and following up acceptors. In these cases, training should be aimed at providing them with sound knowledge and a full understanding of the characteristics of these drugs so that they will be able to:

—describe them to lay people in simple words, paying particular attention to menstrual disturbances, since these are by far the most common complaint and reason for discontinuation;

—identify contraindications or conditions that require medical supervision;

—instruct users so that they can recognize side-effects and conditions requiring immediate unscheduled return to the clinic;

—recognize complications and decide when referrals are necessary;

—keep appropriate records of admission and follow-up data on patients; and

—supervise the work of others for whom they are responsible.

In addition to the knowledge and skills described above, health workers who are to provide injectables also need to know how to communicate with the client and others who may be involved. The subjects to be covered in training in communication with the client should include:

—how to establish good rapport with clients initially so that they trust the health worker;

—how to ensure that the client fully understands what is involved in the choice and use of the method;

—how to assist the client and her partner in making the decision that is best for them;

—the potential importance of the views of other significant family members and how to help the client deal with them;

—how to encourage an amicable resolution of any differences between the client and the health service; and

—how to arrange for follow-up, with the cooperation of the client.

Both *sound knowledge* and *good communication techniques* are essential if the method is to be appropriately promoted and the risk of discontinuation as a result either of ignorance or unnecessary anxiety is to be reduced. Trainers should be able to present the relevant information:

(1) clearly, and without jargon or excessively technical language; (2) concisely, limiting the material to what is essential and avoiding anything that is highly technical or academic in character. Questions, particularly about the disadvantages of the method, should be dealt with honestly and fully; health workers should be encouraged to ask the trainer questions and the latter should employ good listening techniques so that the anxieties of the health worker can be dealt with. In addition, materials should be provided which can be used by the health worker in communicating with the client and her family. Role-playing and modelling are two simple and effective techniques that can be used in training.

Lay workers

Many programmes owe much of their success to the efforts of voluntary workers. Volunteers can include both lay workers and trained health professionals. Programme managers who wish to make use of voluntary help must specify clearly defined roles and tasks for volunteers and the lines of responsibility.

Volunteers have been shown to be particularly useful for:

—motivating and recruiting new acceptors;

—giving information and advice;

—assisting with the follow-up of users.

Training courses

Trainers should have appropriate field experience and be skilled in teaching and communicating. A 1- or 2-day training course for health workers or volunteers should include the following:

—a lecture on injectable contraceptives (definition, mode of action, medical aspects);

—a demonstration of, and practical experience in giving injectables (for health personnel);

—instruction on the counselling of users and a demonstration of information materials;

—instruction in reporting and recording information, using a check-list;

—instruction on how to supervise other workers.

It should not be necessary to acquire additional teaching materials or equipment other than those used for general training in family planning. However, hand-outs or information leaflets specifically describing injectables and how they are used in the programme should be produced.

Trainees should be followed up to ensure that their knowledge and skill in providing injectable contraceptives are maintained.

Check-list

A check-list appropriate to local needs can be used by non-physicians for the purpose of screening for contra-indications to the use of injectables among potential acceptors. It may also be used during follow-up to identify side-effects or complications (see pages 69–71). A check-list is also a useful teaching aid since it helps to underline important points. Trainees should be shown how it can be used and understand its limitations.

Costs

Training costs may include:

—travelling costs for trainers and trainees;

—living allowance for trainers and trainees;

—hire of premises, e.g., local village hall;

—hire of equipment, e.g., projector, video recorder;

—honorarium for trainers;

—printing costs of information materials.

Possible sources of funding for training are given in Annex 2.

8. Evaluation

Definition and purposes of evaluation

Evaluation is the process of systematically collecting and analysing information about a specific programme or activity in order to analyse its effectiveness and to decide about possible courses of action for the future. Simply stated, evaluation in programmes using injectables is aimed at improving current activities and services and in assisting the programme manager in planning for the future. Evaluation is therefore a decision-making tool and an integral part of the managerial process for programme development and implementation.

The information obtained through evaluation should immediately be used by service providers, administrators and communities to develop the delivery and acceptability of long-acting contraceptives. Thus, evaluation should lead to:

—improved service delivery procedures;

—further development of supply and logistics systems;

—more effective education of the client either through the mass media or through staff–client contact;

—improved performance of both technical and managerial staff;

—strengthened staff supervision; and

—improved linkage and coordination between governmental, nongovernmental and private sector providers.

Evaluation helps managers to develop the injectable contraceptive services in a rational and systematic manner. While the conclusions drawn from an evaluation exercise are valuable in themselves, the evaluation process as such may be just as important and useful because it often forces the manager to observe the service more closely. This, in turn, is likely to lead to improved understanding and a more constructive and flexible approach to future programming decisions.

The evaluation process

The process of evaluation consists of the following five steps:

—identifying the subject(s) for evaluation;

—developing a plan or design for carrying out the evaluation;

—implementing the evaluation;

—analysing the findings;

—using the findings in problem-solving and improving services.

Because evaluation is an integral part of the managerial process, the development and implementation of an evaluation scheme should proceed hand in hand with the planning and implementation of the injectable contraceptive service itself.

Programme managers are responsible for evaluation, regardless of their level of overall responsibility.

The local clinic director, the district supervisor, and the national programme manager should all perceive evaluation as part of their duties. In subsequent sections of this chapter, some of the topics and indicators that may concern programme managers at different levels will be discussed.

Evaluation schemes vary in complexity depending on the nature of the programme being evaluated, the availability of time and resources, and the degree of sophistication and training of the personnel carrying out the evaluation. The programme manager should not hesitate to call upon those trained in evaluation methodology to assist in the design and implementation of evaluation schemes. For a more complete introduction to the principles and methods of evaluation, see the additional sources of information at the end of this chapter.

Topics for evaluation and performance indicators

The information provided here on performance indicators is not intended to be exhaustive but merely to indicate the types of data on programme performance that the programme manager is likely to find of value. The final selection of topics for evaluation and of indicators of performance will depend on what the programme manager considers to be important for future decisions and planning.

Prevalence

This is the number or percentage of women of reproductive age who are currently using injectable contraceptives. Surveys are the usual means of obtaining data on prevalence. These are available for many countries, e.g., from the World Fertility Survey series and studies carried out in collaboration with the Centers for Disease Control and Westinghouse Health Systems.[a] When studies are conducted before and after injectables are introduced, managers can compare the prevalence rates and thus determine whether the method has been well received and is successful. They can also compare rates for injectables with those for other types of contraceptive to see whether they have become more widely accepted since the programme began.

---

[a] MONTEITH, R. ET AL. *Studies in family planning*, **12**: 331–340 (1981).

Programme performance indicators

Programme performance indicators are standard statistical indices or measures that allow managers to review levels, trends, and changes in service outputs and characteristics over time.

These help the manager to answer such questions as: Is the programme operating at the desired level of output? Is it serving the appropriate client population? How are clients referred for services? Why do clients choose injectables? How many clients discontinue after a given period of time?

Data for certain programme indicators are easily collected, tabulated, and analysed on a routine, continuous basis. Some of the most frequently used indicators of performance of injectable contraceptives are described below.

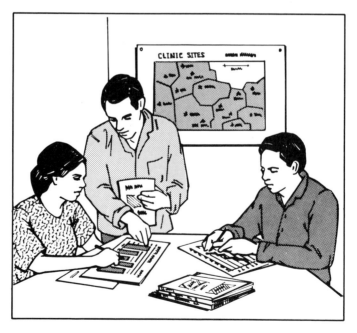

Fig. 10. Data on programme performance should be collected and analysed on a regular basis.

Number of new acceptors of injectables. Simple tabulations can be done by month, quarter, year, or other standard reporting period. Figures can easily be displayed in the form of bar charts or line graphs.

Number of users continuing after given periods of time. Since injectable contraceptives are given at 2- or 3-monthly intervals, it is useful to know how many are still using the method after 3, 6 or 12 months.

Number of users discontinuing the method after given periods of time. The number of discontinuations is usually reported for 12-monthly intervals. It can be calculated by subtracting the number of users continuing to use the method after 12 months from the sum total of the number of acceptors at the start of the 12-months plus the number of new acceptors over the 12-month period.

Frequency of reasons cited for discontinuing at various periods, with particular emphasis on bleeding disturbances. Because bleeding disturbances account for a significant number of discontinuations in some countries, programme managers should ensure that service providers record all reports by clients of menstrual disturbances, as well as other side-effects, such as weight gain or headaches.

Age of the client. This statistic can be expressed either as the average age of clients in a standard reporting period, or as the distribution of clients over a series of age intervals (e.g., 25–29, 30–34, etc.).

Number of living children of the client. Expressed as an average, this statistic is important because it helps managers to assess the effect of the programme on fertility patterns and its demographic impact. In some countries, it may be necessary to distinguish between male and female living children.

Primary information sources. This is a tabulation of clients according to the source of information that was most important in their decision to use injectables. The figures will allow managers to identify the most effective methods of information and education. Sources might be classified as: (*a*) friends, relatives, and neighbours; (*b*) the media (e.g., radio, television, newspapers, other printed materials); (*c*) programme personnel (e.g., field workers, clinic personnel, community distribution agents); (*d*) other health personnel (e.g., non-programme health workers, private practitioners); (*e*) other. Such a classification can, of course, be modified in accordance with local programme characteristics.

The above performance indicators can easily be derived from the family planning record forms of users of injectables. Thus, each form serves not only as the official history of use of injectables for medical and legal purposes and future reference, but also as the source document for programme monitoring.

Non-routine studies and surveys

In addition to the routine and continuous monitoring of basic service statistics in order to assess whether programmes are developing satisfactorily, more sophisticated programme evaluation exercises are occasionally needed to make more refined analyses and to modify programme design so as to achieve better results. Some of the major types of studies relevant to injectables are discussed briefly below. Introductory trials are discussed on pages 95–98.

Client characteristics. Studies are frequently designed to identify the characteristics of the clients served by programmes so that a clearer picture of the women they tend to attract can be obtained. The characteristics that can be studied in this way include occupation, income, place of residence, religion, and level of education. Such studies can often easily be carried out by using data obtained from client medical record forms or from interviews conducted before or after the use of injectables has been started. Occasional studies of client characteristics complement the routine analysis of basic service statistics.

Client satisfaction. A major area of concern regarding the use of injectables in family planning programmes is the degree of client satisfaction with the method. This can be measured in terms of the number who continue or reuse the method, the frequency of discontinuation and the reasons cited for discontinuing. Dissatisfied clients can have a serious impact on programme performance. Abnormally high rates of discontinuation often indicate poor client screening, counselling, or management of side-effects. Client satisfaction can easily be assessed at the time of follow-up visits, or over the longer term through special surveys carried out by means of home visits or mailed questionnaires, depending on the literacy of the population served.

Knowledge and attitudes of clients and providers. Evaluation of knowledge and attitudes about injectables can be extremely important in identifying fears, misinformation, rumours, and other influences hindering their acceptance. Having identified such factors, programme managers can design information strategies to correct false impressions and unfavourable attitudes. Because service providers sometimes oppose or resist programmes providing injectable contraceptives, it is important to assess their knowledge and attitudes as well as those of potential clients. Knowledge and attitude surveys are important not only among providers and clients, but also in the community in general.

Availability and accessibility of services. Unavailability or limited availability of services can be a major obstacle to injectable programmes. Several factors may be involved in this issue. Policies and legal regulations on age, parity, consent, and medical personnel may have an impact on the availability of services and client eligibility. In addition, the number and location of service sites and the type of service delivery channels can affect accessibility. Studies of all these factors are often of great importance when programmes are being planned or modified.

Programme design. Different types of service delivery systems, information and education programmes, client referral systems, and client flow systems can affect the efficiency, effectiveness, and cost of injectable contraceptive services. It is important, therefore, to evaluate programme design features, especially when modifications are being considered. Conducting a small pilot or demonstration project is a useful way of evaluating programme design before implementing it on a large scale.

Cost-effectiveness. Very little is known about the total costs of injectable contraceptive services, or about the cost-effectiveness of various delivery systems or information and education approaches (e.g., word-of-mouth as compared with mass media). Precise cost studies can be difficult, since they involve sophisticated cost-accounting techniques, but are essential in determining the most efficient programme design.

Other indicators. A list of other indicators that can be used in the evaluation of services is given in Annex 5.

Additional sources of information

For the reader interested in a more comprehensive treatment of the general principles and methodologies of programme evaluation that can be applied to programming and managerial decision-making, the following publications are especially recommended:

Health programme evaluation: guiding principles for its application in the managerial process for national health development. Geneva, World Health Organization, 1981 ("Health for All" Series, No. 6).

REYNOLDS, J. ET AL. *Evaluation handbook for family planning programs.* Rockville, MD, United States Department of Health, Education, and Welfare, 1978.

9. Operational and other research

The introduction of a new contraceptive method into family planning programmes raises a number of questions. For example, how can the acceptability and effectiveness of the method in a specific society and in others of similar characteristics be adequately evaluated? What measures should be adopted to ensure user satisfaction and compliance in the use of the method? How can this knowledge be obtained so that it will be useful for programme planners and policy makers?

Introductory trials

The main purpose of introductory trials is to assess, through a limited initial cohort of users, both problems and user needs in a programme situation. From such studies, service norms and counselling procedures can be established for use in the national programme.

Objectives

Introductory trials are the first service-based evaluations of a contraceptive method. Their objective is to facilitate the wide-scale introduction and registration of the product. They provide information on use–effectiveness, continuation rates, actual side-effects, and adverse health events. They are usually undertaken on groups of 1000–10 000 users. The introductory trial plays a critical role in fostering acceptance of the method, not only among the population served by the clinic but also among the health care providers. It provides an opportunity for staff unfamiliar with the method to learn by experience about its inherent side-effects, and the clinical and counselling issues that may arise with its use. It gives staff the opportunity to deal with their own potential biases for or against the method through direct observation of the user population's perceptions of the method. It also allows the providers to understand the impact of the service delivery system on the acceptability of the method and to explore mechanisms that could serve to improve clinic services, in relation not only to the specific method, but to the family planning programme as a whole.

The development of introductory trials entails three phases: planning; implementation and monitoring; and analysis and recommendations. Planning begins with preparation of a protocol and of forms for recording essential data. The forms should have a simple format and be suitable for a service-delivery setting. They should address: admission information, when subjects returned for injections, reasons for discontinuation, pregnancy and rare adverse effects. In addition, a medical selection criteria check-list, a manual on completion of forms, and a counselling check-list should be developed. An informed consent form should also be prepared to cover the major points in the Declaration of Helsinki on protection of rights of human subjects. This will ensure that study volunteers are aware that they are participating in a study to evaluate the contraceptive and that they have been informed of the risks and benefits of their participation.

Appropriate informational and educational materials for both users and providers should be developed and tested prior to the study. These materials should be modified and updated as experience is gained in the study. Orientation and training for staff participating in the project should include a detailed description of the method, how it works, its advantages and disadvantages in comparison with other methods offered in the clinic, the management of side-effects, techniques for counselling potential acceptors and for addressing questions and concerns arising during use of the method, the use of informational materials for accept-ors in the counselling session, procedures for reviewing and submitting case record forms, maintaining a logbook, and techniques for locating users and reminding them about missed follow-up visits. Since the introductory trial is designed to see how the method can be incorporated into the normal routine of the clinic and to determine how many people are interested in using this method when they have a range of choices, the staff must be trained to explain the method in a similar manner as for the other methods provided by the clinic.

Regular monitoring visits should be made by the study coordinator. These visits permit the assessment of all activities carried out at the clinic in relation to the method, including initial counselling, data collection, and action in regard to medical issues. Problems encountered should be reviewed on site and solutions sought. Periodic meetings of investigators should be held, at which the investigators can talk about the problems and queries that have arisen and share their experiences and ideas on possible solutions with their colleagues.

Plans should be made for adequate and timely interim analysis of data generated from the study to allow plans to be made for registration and widespread distribution of the product. All data should be reported to the drug regulatory agency as available so that registration of the product can be expedited. On completion of the introductory trial, a meeting should be held between officials of the Ministry of Health, principal investigators, and other relevant parties at which the findings of the study are reviewed. Where appropriate, information based on the results of the study may subsequently be incorporated into package inserts, informational materials, etc.

Design aspects

Investigators planning to assess the performance of a new method should also weigh carefully the most appropriate research design, especially if case–control or comparative studies are envisaged. Furthermore, the design of forms and questionnaires should take into account the most important variables relating to the method, especially known side-effects and their outcomes. In the case of injectable contraceptives, one reason to stop using them can be "irregular menstrual bleeding", but it is also

97

important to know what impact this side-effect may be having on the woman's family or sexual relations. When use is discontinued for "personal" reasons, an attempt should be made to obtain additional information. Despite the many possible ramifications of the reasons for method discontinuation, it is recommended that the study forms should be kept simple and the questions reduced to the essential minimum.

Development of new injectable contraceptives

It is estimated that over 6 million women around the world are currently using injectable preparations and implantable devices for fertility regulation; of these, at least two-thirds are using DMPA. However, it is generally believed that the popularity of such methods would be considerably increased if they were further improved so that bleeding irregularities—the commonest cause of discontinuation—were avoided.

In an attempt to minimize the vaginal bleeding and disturbances associated with progestogen-only approaches to contraception, work is being undertaken by WHO on progestogen/estrogen combinations given as monthly injections. These have the potential advantages of high contraceptive effectiveness, good cycle control and rapid return of fertility combined with the logistic and cultural advantages of all injectable contraceptives, namely that they can be administered by non-physicians in rural areas. The major disadvantage, both for users and for family planning programmes, is that a clinic visit is necessary every 30 days.

Additional sources of information

KAZI, A. ET AL. Phase IV study of the injection Norigest in Pakistan. *Contraception*, **32**: 395–403 (1985).

RAHMAN, S. S. ET AL. Introduction of the injectable contraceptive NET-EN into family planning clinics in Bangladesh. *Bulletin of the World Health Organization*, **63**: 785–791 (1985).

MEADE, C. W. ET AL. A clinical study of norethisterone enantate in rural Mexico. *Studies in family planning*, **15**: 143–148 (1984).

Multinational comparative trial of long-acting injectable contraceptives: norethisterone enantate given in two dosage regimens and depot-medroxyprogesterone acetate. Final report. *Contraception*, **28**: 1–20 (1983).

Annex 1. Countries and territories in which DMPA and NET-EN are registered

In 1989, DMPA was registered in the following countries and territories for use for contraception:

Afghanistan
Angola
Antigua
Bahrain
Bangladesh
Barbados
Belgium
Bermuda
Bolivia
Cameroon
Colombia
Costa Rica
Côte d'Ivoire
Curacao
Cyprus
Denmark
Dominican Republic
Ecuador
Egypt
El Salvador
Ethiopia
France
Germany, Federal
  Republic of
Ghana
Greece
Guatemala
Guyana
Haiti
Honduras

Hong Kong
Iceland
Indonesia
Iraq
Israel
Jamaica
Kenya
Kuwait
Lebanon
Liberia
Libyan Arab
  Jamahiriya
Madagascar
Malawi
Malaysia
Mexico
Morocco
Myanmar
Netherlands
New Zealand
Nicaragua
Nigeria
Norway
Pakistan
Panama
Peru
Portugal
Qatar
Republic of
  Korea

Réunion
Rwanda
Saudi Arabia
Sierra Leone
Singapore
South Africa
Spain
Sri Lanka
Sudan
Suriname
Sweden
Switzerland
Syrian Arab
  Republic
Thailand
Trinidad
Turkey
Uganda
United Arab
  Emirates
United Kingdom
United Republic
  of Tanzania
Uruguay
Venezuela
Yugoslavia
Zaire
Zimbabwe

In 1989 NET-EN was registered in the following countries and territories for use for contraception:

Antigua and
  Barbuda
Australia
Bahamas
Bangladesh
Barbados
Belize
Benin
Burkina Faso
Burundi
Cape Verde
Central African
  Republic
Chad
Congo
Costa Rica
Côte d'Ivoire
Denmark
Dominica
Dominican Republic

El Salvador
Fiji
France
Germany, Federal
  Republic of
Ghana
Grenada
Guinea
Guinea-Bissau
Guyana
India
Indonesia
Kenya
Madagascar
Malawi
Malaysia
Mali
Mexico
Mozambique
New Zealand

Niger
Nigeria
Oman
Pakistan
Peru
Philippines
Portugal
Rwanda
Saint Lucia
Singapore
South Africa
Spain
Sri Lanka
Swaziland
Thailand
Togo
Uganda
United Kingdom
Zambia
Zimbabwe

Annex 2. International sources of technical and funding assistance for injectable contraceptive programmes

The following is a selective listing of governmental, intergovernmental and private organizations that provide funding and/or technical assistance for family planning programmes. For more extensive listings and detailed descriptions of the work of the various organizations, see *Guide to sources of international population assistance 1985*, New York, United Nations Fund for Population Activities, 1985.

The Asia Foundation,
P.O. Box 3223,
San Francisco, CA, USA

and

2301 E street N.W.,
Washington, DC 20037, USA

The D.K. Tyagi Fund,
Suite 800,
875 Sixth Avenue,
New York, NY 10001, USA

Family Health International (FHI),
One Triangle Drive,
Research Triangle Park,
NC 27709, USA

International Committee on Management of Population
  Programmes (ICOMP),
158 Jalan Dahlia,
Taman Uda Jaya,
68000 Ampang,
Kuala Lumpur,
Malaysia

Family Planning International Assistance (FPIA),
810 Seventh Avenue,
New York, NY 10019, USA

International Planned Parenthood Federation (IPPF),
Regents College,
Inner Circle,
Regents Park,
London NW1 4NS,
England

Japanese Organization for International Cooperation in
  Family Planning (JOICFP),
Hoken Kaikan Bekkan,
1-1 Sadohara-cho, Ichigaya,
Shinjuku-ku, Tokyo 162,
Japan

The Pathfinder Fund,
1330 Boylston Street,
Chestnut Hill,
Boston, MA 02167, USA

Population Crisis Committee (PCC) and the Draper Fund,
1200 19th Street, NW,
Washington, DC 20036, USA

Population Services Europe (PSE),
108 Whitfield Street,
London W1P 6BE,
England

Program for Appropriate Technology in Health,
PATH Building,
4 Nickerson Street,
Seattle, WA 98109, USA

World Neighbors,
5116 North Portland Avenue,
Oklahoma City, OK, USA

Annex 3. Principal manufacturers of injectable contraceptives

DMPA

- Upjohn SA, 2670 Puurs, Belgium.
  Product: medroxyprogesterone acetate in sterile aqueous suspension; 1-ml vials, 10-ml vials, and 1-ml syringes, containing 150 mg/ml; 3-ml vials containing 50 mg/ml.

- Farmitalia Carlo Erba, Via Imbonati 24, 20159 Milan, Italy.
  Product: medroxyprogesterone acetate in sterile aqueous suspension; 3-ml vials containing 50 mg/ml.

- Organon International BV, P.O. Box 20, 5340 BH Oss, The Netherlands.
  Product: medroxyprogesterone acetate in sterile aqueous suspension; 1-ml vials containing 150 mg/ml.

Several companies in Indonesia and Thailand also manufacture DMPA for local use.

NET-EN

- Schering AG, P.O. Box 650311, Mullerstrasse 170–178, Berlin (West).
  Product: norethisterone enantate in non-aqueous oily solution; 1-ml ampoules and 1-ml syringes containing 200 mg/ml.

- Gideon Richter Ltd, 1103 Budapest, Hungary.
  Product: norethisterone enantate in non-aqueous oily solution; 1-ml ampoules containing 200 mg/ml.

Annex 4. Calculation of the equilibrium level

The number of users of a particular method of contraception at the end of any given year is equal to the number of users at the beginning of the year together with the number of new acceptors (N), less the number of users who drop out during the year. To simplify this model, the number of new acceptors in the long term (equilibrium) is assumed to be based on the number of women who become eligible for contraceptive use (for example, those entering childbearing age) and the relative acceptability of the method. The total number who discontinue is assumed to be a percentage of all users of the method in the programme in the year in question, and is based on the number of women leaving the fertile age group, the percentage of women desiring another child (related to average birth spacing), the percentage of women who experience medical problems with the method, and the percentage who discontinue for other or unspecified reasons. The discontinuation rate (D) can be estimated by means of a pilot project, or from data acquired in other countries. As will be seen, the equilibrium number of users (E) is sensitive to both the discontinuation rate and to the yearly number of new acceptors.

A simple mathematical relationship exists between the equilibrium number of users, the discontinuation rate, and the yearly number of new acceptors (for simplicity, this number, N, is taken as constant, i.e., population growth is assumed to be zero, and the relative acceptability of the method to remain constant). If D is expressed as a percentage, then:

$$E = K \times N,$$

where the factor $K = (100 - D)/D$.

The relationship between D and the factor K is shown in Table A4.1.

Table A4.1. Relationship between discontinuation rate and factor K

12-month discontinuation rate (D) (%)	K
10	9.0
20	4.0
30	2.33
40	1.50
50	1.00
60	0.67
70	0.43
80	0.25
90	0.11

These relationships can also be used to find the number of new acceptors needed to maintain a target equilibrium number of users if the discontinuation rate is known. This is given by $N = E/K$.

Effect of varying numbers of acceptors

Fig. A4.1 shows that, for a discontinuation rate of 30% per year, different equilibrium levels are reached if different numbers of women accept the method each year. In programme A, 100 000 new women per year adopt the method, and the programme achieves a steady state or equilibrium level of approximately 233 000 users. Programme B adds 200 000 new acceptors every year, and reaches equilibrium at about 467 000 users. It is important to note that, for any given discontinuation rate, the number of users in the long term is directly proportional to the number of new acceptors. The equilibrium level (or alternatively, the point corresponding to 90% of the ultimate level) is reached at the same time for both programmes.

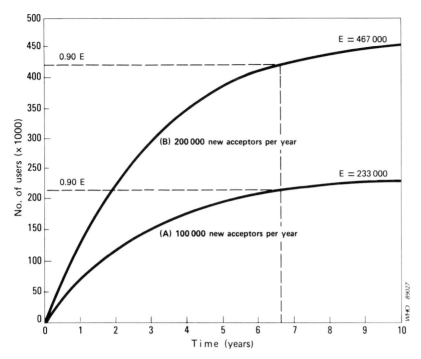

Fig. A4.1. Increase in number of users over time with an annual discontinuation rate of 30%.

Effect of discontinuation

Fig. A4.2 shows the great effect of the discontinuation rate on the equilibrium number of users. Programmes A, B, and C all gain new acceptors at the rate of 200 000 per year, but their users have different discontinuation rates. Programme B (shown by the same curve as in Fig. A4.1) has a discontinuation rate of 30%, yielding an equilibrium user level of 467 000. Programme A has a somewhat higher discontinuation rate of 40%, and reaches equilibrium at 300 000 users—36% lower than B. Programme C has a lower discontinuation rate of 20%, which yields an ultimate equilibrium level of 800 000 users—71% more than Programme B. Quite clearly, this is an effect that managers should be aware of.

A second effect of discontinuation rates is also illustrated by Fig. A4.2. The time required to reach equilibrium is

107

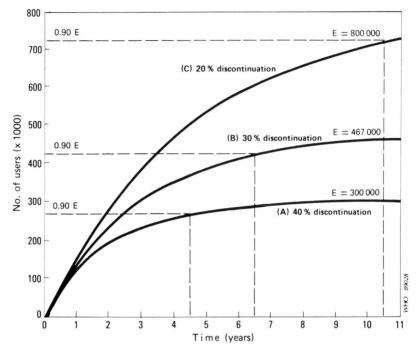

Fig. A4.2. Effect of discontinuation rates on number of users, for a constant number of new acceptors (200 000 per year).

shortest for the programme with the highest discontinuation rate. Looking at the time required to reach 90% of the number of users in the steady state, we find that the programme with the 40% discontinuation rate takes approximately 4.5 years, the programme with a discontinuation rate of 30% takes 6.5 years, and that with a discontinuation rate of 20% takes 10.5 years. These times are independent of the rate at which new acceptors are added.

The initial effort

The relationships illustrated in Fig. A4.1 and A4.2 are independent of the initial numbers of users in a programme. This fact has a marked bearing on the strategy

108

to be used in the introductory phase. As already noted, the time needed to achieve a steady number of users can be several years, depending on the discontinuation rate, on the assumption that the number of new acceptors remains constant throughout the programme. To reduce this time, programme planners might wish to enlist a higher number of new acceptors during the first few years of the programme. When a new method is being introduced, there may be an initial high demand for it from women who wish to use contraception but have been unable or unwilling to use any previously available method. More typically, however, a substantial effort has to be made to attract new users to an unfamiliar method. This is costly in terms of personnel, training, informational materials and supplies.

In general, the greater the effort that can be made, the faster an equilibrium level of users can be attained. However, there are pitfalls in the decision-making process which can have profound effects on logistics management, as illustrated in Fig. A4.3.

All the curves shown in Fig. A4.3 represent new contraceptive programmes, all of which are expected to have a 30% annual discontinuation rate and a steady-state addition of 200 000 new acceptors per year, resulting in a long-term user level of 467 000.

Curve B represents the same programme as before, in which 200 000 new acceptors are added each year from the beginning of the programme, so that the 90% equilibrium level is reached in around 6.5 years.

The planners of the programme represented by curve C are dissatisfied with the long time taken to reach equilibrium, and propose a 3-year start-up period in which 500 000 new acceptors are added each year. This requires vastly increased staffing, and also the procurement and storage of a much larger supply of contraceptives for these 3 years. At the end of the start-up period, the programme will have enrolled around 750 000 women and the level of effort is then reduced so that only 200 000 new acceptors per year are added. Because of the effect of discontinuation, after several years the number of users will fall to close to the equilibrium level of 467 000. Thus a large, costly initial effort produces only a transient effect.

Curve A represents a programme where the planners believe that a start-up phase having only a modestly higher

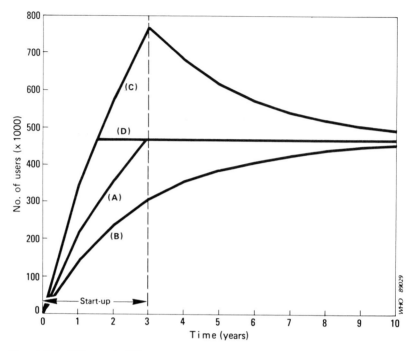

Fig. A4.3. Effect of different start-up phase targets on user equilibrium level.

target of 300 000 new acceptors per year could be implemented at an acceptable cost. Equilibrium would be achieved in 3 years with no wasted effort.

The planners of programme C have the option of cutting off the start-up phase after $1\frac{1}{2}$ years when the equilibrium level is reached, as shown by curve D. This would reduce the total cost of the start-up phase, but does not avoid the need for a large increase in staff and much larger supplies of materials for this short period.

Once the above parameters have been determined, forecasting of materials requirements for injectables is straightforward. Supplies of injectables must be available continuously for women already enrolled in the programme, as well as for new acceptors.

Annex 5. Additional indicators for evaluating injectable contraceptive services

The indicators listed here are additional to those already discussed in Chapter 8. Indicators of efficiency, effectiveness and impact will not be required until the new contraceptive method has been in use for a sufficient period of time. The status of programme implementation should be confirmed through the use of selected indicators of relevance, adequacy and progress. A variety of evaluation methods may be required, including in-depth case studies.

Indicators

A. *Of relevance/adequacy*   *Evaluation method*

    1. Policy support—do population or   Case study
    health policies exist which provide
    a mandate for introducing injectable
    contraceptives?

    2. *Programme planning*—is the injectables   Case study
    programme or strategy supported by a
    plan which contains:

      —a quantified definition of the health
      or social problems to be addressed?
      —quantified objectives of health
      improvement and service targets to be
      achieved within a stated time period?
      —a description and size of the particular
      target population to be served?
      —a clear description of the programme
      and its operational strategy?

—a timetable for a plan of action,
indicating the activities to be carried
out in order to introduce injectable
contraceptives and the responsible
units or offices?

3. *Resource generation*—is there evidence   Case study
of appropriate support for the new
services such as:

—budgetary provision for the
additional expenses required to set
up and operate the injectable services?
—external support (technical advice,
information, training, supplies,
financing)?
—cooperation with other governmental
agencies?

B. *Of progress*

1. *Policy revision*—if policies or regulations need revision for implementation   Case study
of the injectable contraceptive strategy,
have appropriate revised texts been
drafted, reviewed, approved, and
enacted?

2. *Procedures development*—have support   Case study
systems and procedures needed to
provide the injectable services been
designed and documented? Specifically:

—have technical guidelines and
instructions for service staff been
drafted, tested and published?
—have clinic recording and reporting
procedures and forms been designed,
tested and documented?
—have monitoring and supervision
procedures for mid-level service
managers been designed, tested and
documented?
—have procedures for client follow-up,
recall and referral been designed and
documented?

—have procurement and distribution procedures for supplies of injectable hormonal contraceptives been worked out and incorporated in the medical supplies system?

3. *Training*—have steps been taken to prepare service staff and managers to deliver injectable contraceptives, as follows:

    Monitoring, case study and survey

—has an in-service training programme been drawn up and materials prepared and tested?
—have the necessary number of training institutions and trainers been selected and prepared?
—have the targeted number of training courses been held as scheduled?
—have the targeted number of service staff and managers of each type received training?
—do the targeted number of service points (facilities) have the trained staff necessary to provide injectable contraceptives continuously?

4. *Information*—have public information messages, methods and materials about injectable contraceptives been developed, tested and used?

    Case study, monitoring

C. *Of service efficiency*

1. *Coverage*—are injectable contraceptives accessible to women of childbearing age? This can be evaluated by:

    Monitoring, survey

—the number of service points that can provide injectable contraceptives;
—the proportion of the population with access to services (e.g., who live within 10 km of a service point);

113

—the proportion of women of
childbearing age aware that injectable
contraceptives are available;
—the percentage of all government
services offering injectables;
—the percentage of districts and towns
in which injectable services are
available;
—the number of days or hours per
week in which the injectable service
is offered in each type of facility.

2. *Output*—how many injectable contraceptives have been provided over a
certain period? This can be evaluated
by:

    Monitoring

—the number of first consultations about
injectables;
—the number of continuing users
(6 months or more);
—the number of injections administered.

3. *Quality*—for what proportion of clients
are the following adequately performed?

    Monitoring,
survey

—history taking;
—preliminary examination;
—record-keeping;
—sterilization of apparatus;
—administration of injections;
—counselling on side-effects;
—monitoring, follow-up;
—injection at appropriate intervals.

4. *Organization*—has the service
administering the injectable programme
been adequately organized? This can be
evaluated by:

    Monitoring,
survey

—the number of referrals from peripheral
service levels;
—the proportion of defaulters followed up
to ascertain the reason for their failure
to attend;

—the activities and support provided by other agencies and sectors, and by communities for establishing and maintaining the programme;

—the completeness and accuracy of patient records.

5. *Management of supplies*—on an individual facility basis. This can be evaluated by:

Monitoring, survey

—the number of days' supply of injectable hormonal contraceptives available;
—the monthly usage rate over the previous year;
—the adequacy of the supply records;
—the expiry date on current stock;
—a history of continuous supply without interruptions caused by stocks becoming exhausted.

6. *Costs and efficiency*—has resource consumption and its relationship to the delivery of injectable services been satisfactory? This can be evaluated by:

Monitoring, survey

—the total extra expenditure incurred in setting up and implementing the service, by type of expenditure and time period;
—the cost per acceptor and acceptor-year;
—the ratio of acceptors to trained staff;
—the output of newly introduced, related services (cervical smears, self-administered breast examination, home-based mother's record);
—the staff attitude towards the use of injectables

D. *Of programme effectiveness*

1. *Family planning prevalence*—the effect of the programme on

Monitoring, survey

115

contraceptive use. This can be evaluated by:

—the number of clients continuing to use injectable contraceptives after 6, 12, 18 and 24 months;
—the frequency of reasons cited for discontinuing at various periods;
—the number of couple–years of protection provided by injectables;
—the overall prevalence of contraceptive use before and after the introduction of injectables;
—changes in method prevalence rates;
—the characteristics of users of injectable contraceptives, e.g., age, family size, education, income level.

2. *Efficacy*—as reflected by the following contraceptive failure rates (pregnancy rates):

Monitoring, survey

—annual;
—per 100 woman–years of use;
—per 100 acceptors.

3. *Side-effects*—as shown by the percentage of users who report:

Monitoring, survey

—amenorrhoea;
—menstrual disturbances;
—weight gain;
—headaches, nausea, nervousness;
—effect on lactation;
—ectopic pregnancies.

4. *Client satisfaction*—as expressed by:

Monitoring, survey

—the percentage of clients who will continue or reuse the method;
—the percentage of clients who would recommend the method to friends;
—the reasons for dissatisfaction and the frequency with which they are cited.

E. *Impact*

Monitoring, survey

After several years and wide acceptance of the injectable service, it may be
of value to attempt to measure the
impact of the programme on such
indicators as:

—overall fertility rate;
—infant mortality rate;
—maternal mortality rate;
—pregnancy rate by parity and age;
—birth interval by age group;
—percentage of unwanted pregnancies;
—abortion rate (spontaneous and
  induced);
—complications of induced abortions;
—complications of pregnancy.